A DOCTOR'S LOOK AT LIFE AND HISTORY

A Doctor's Look at Life and History

by

David S. Muckle, *M.B., B.S., F.R.C.S.*

ORIEL PRESS

First printed in Great Britain, 1970

ISBN 0 85362 089 X
Library of Congress Catalog Card Number

Published by Oriel Press Limited
at 32 Ridley Place, Newcastle upon Tyne, England. NE1 8LH.
Text set in 11 on 13 point Baskerville
Printed in Great Britain by
Northumberland Press Limited, Gateshead

CONTENTS

ILLUSTRATIONS

ACKNOWLEDGEMENT

I wish to acknowledge my gratitude to Margaret Stevenson who typed the articles and gave such excellent advice, to Bruce Allsopp and Ronnie Adams whose encouragement was invaluable.

D.S.M.

FAMOUS PEOPLE—FAMOUS DISEASES

HUMAN DISEASES fascinate most people, but never more so than when they can be identified with the famous. The inborn metabolic disorder (porphyrinuria) of George III that led to his periodic bouts of insanity and abdominal pain, the megalomania of Hitler from the tertiary stage of syphilis, the rickets and hump-back of Alexander Pope that reduced his height to four feet six inches, made ridiculous his amorous advances to Lady Mary Wortley Montague and made him ultra-sensitive to society as a whole, the neurosis of Charles Darwin, now thought to be part of the general ill health of Chaga's disease (a condition of infectious origin due to a small organism in the blood, the organism being transmitted by an insect bite and endemic in armadillos and other South American animals he studied on his *Beagle* voyage), the throat infection (probably a quinsy or peri-tonsillar abscess) that killed George Washington, the baldness of Queen Elizabeth from congenital syphilis, the hunched form of Richard III, the wart on Cromwell's nose, are as commonly known today as their diseases were to their contemporaries. But of all the famous people and their illnesses, none has aroused such interest in both the medical and lay literature as that of Henry VIII.

Athletic and handsome, an able sportsman, a poet of no mean ability, bluff King Hal; or selfish, ruthless, a tyrant, a madman, obese, foul-smelling ... which is true?

While young, eighteen to be exact, Henry married his

sister-in-law, Catherine of Aragon, whose marriage to Arthur had ended with his premature death from tuberculosis. Their marriage had never been consummated. Catherine had six pregnancies in her second marriage and many miscarriages but all save one, the Princess Mary, ended in stillbirth, abortion or premature death in infancy. Now the House of Tudor required a male heir to secure succession to the throne but at the age of forty-two Catherine ceased to menstruate. Henry, having lived with her for eighteen years and already in love with Anne Boleyn, decided that the final opportunity for a son with Catherine had passed. She had tried continuously over the years but miscarriage after miscarriage had blighted all her efforts. Henry had one son by a mistress, Elizabeth Blount, and had contemplated setting him up as heir. His decision to divorce Catherine was a lengthy business, involving in the end a break with the Roman Church, but, in May 1533, the divorce came through. Henry had already married Anne Boleyn four months before and in September Elizabeth was born. Then followed a series of miscarriages. Henry, despite his long wrangle with the established Church, always regarded himself as a deeply religious man and feared that, because he had previously had a liaison with Anne's sister Mary, his second marriage was as incestuous as his first. Anne, however, more spirited than her predecessor, refused to give up queenship so easily, and Henry was finally forced to resort to the headsman's axe to rid himself of a now detested spouse. This marked the beginning of the period when Henry's actions were founded on pathology of the brain, namely the third stage of syphilis. The repeated miscarriages and child wastage, the thin patchy hair of Mary, her defective vision and peculiarly shaped head and Elizabeth's alopecia, are all signs of congenital syphilitic disease.

Jane Seymour produced a son but died of puerperal fever shortly afterwards, leaving Henry a weak and ailing boy who later became Edward VI (who died in adolescence from tuberculosis). Anne of Cleves was the next marital candidate but the marriage was quickly annulled because of Henry's distaste for her plain face and clumsy body. Catherine Howard soon followed but, like her cousin, Anne Boleyn, went to the block, a victim of court intrigue and the easily aroused anger of the ageing Henry. Finally, in the last years of his life, Catherine Parr was both nurse and companion to the cantankerous old king.

He now measured forty-four inches around the waist and fifty-seven round the chest. His legs were so obese and covered with foul-smelling ulcers (from syphilis) that he was unable to stand and had to be hoisted from room to room with the aid of a pulley.

From a good-natured, fun-loving man and an able king he had changed to a pathological despot under the mental effects of syphilis. The pain from an infection of the bones of his legs and the associate ulcers made him irritable, while an old head injury sustained during jousting caused increasing headaches and loss of concentration. The break with Rome, the dissolution of the monasteries, the abolition of over a hundred hospitals for the poor and sick, the suppression of numerous colleges, all originated from the little spirochaete organism that had multiplied in his brain. What history would be without it we will never know.

Not all cases of insanity are due to infection. It was said of Jean Paul Marat 'he would have drunk blood of his mother from his father's skull'. He was born in the little Swiss Canton village of Boudry in 1743. He had a strong character when young, throwing himself out of a window once into the street as a protest against his father's discipline. He later studied medicine in Paris, Holland and London and obtained an honorary degree at St. Andrews. In 1774 he published his first political book, *Chains of Slavery* and it was designed to secure 'the triumph of liberty in England'. This book typifies the man's complete paranoid character for in it he shows an unswervable belief in the correctness and virtue of his own attitudes and an utter contempt of the 'folly' of others. At first

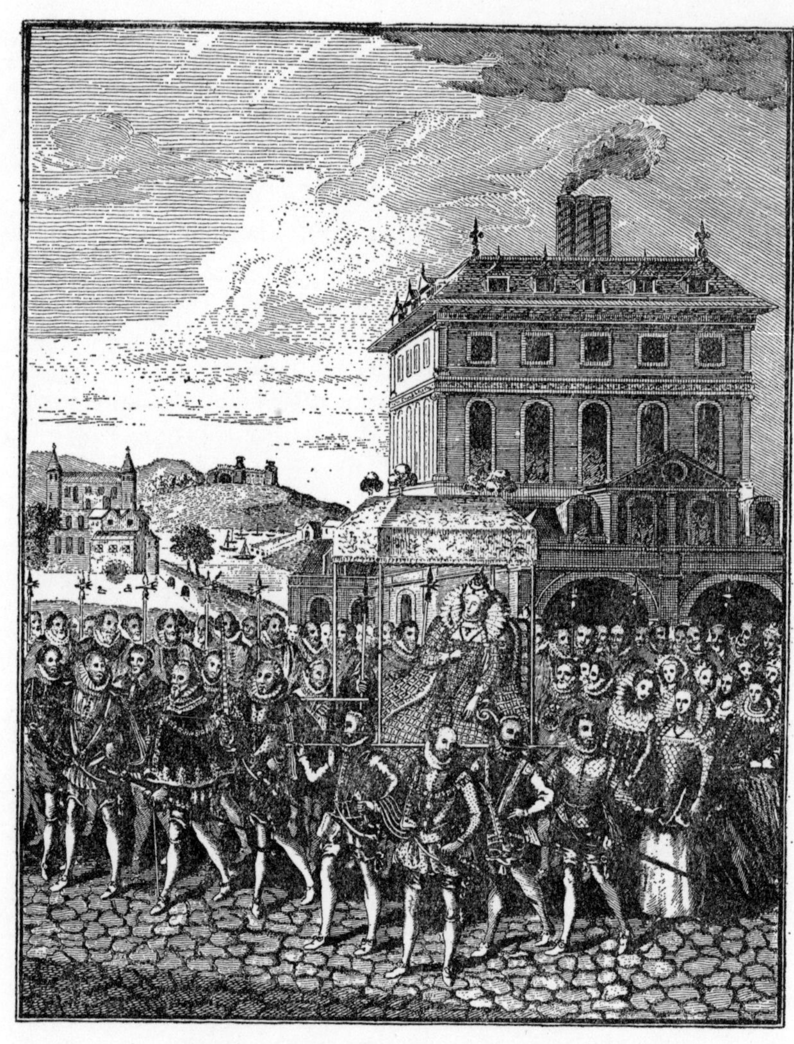

Queen Elizabeth I at Berwick on Tweed

Marat was unable to get this book published and he immediately assumed that there was a deep conspiracy to prevent him from succeeding in medicine and politics. He accepted an appointment with a court aristocrat, while developing fervent revolutionary ideas and publishing pamphlets and columns in the newspaper, *L'Ami du Peuple,* damning the rich and their lucrative ideals. His medical and scientific interests faded away while his influence in the inner circles of the revolution grew. Carlyle states that Marat took part in the attack on the Bastille, although other historians think he is wrong on this point. However, it was Marat's damning orations and inflammatory articles that spread the bitter flames of the French Revolution. He declared that eight hundred gibbets should be erected to hang the 279,000 so-called 'enemies of the Revolution' whose death was necessary to obtain 'la Liberté'.

In the latter part of his life he suffered from increasing delusions of grandeur and an unfortunate skin irritation which produced incessant itching, only relieved by a warm bath. He stated that he had contracted this disease while hiding in the cellars and sewers underground. It was mainly located in the groin and scrotum. Many forms of eczema have been suggested but one of the most likely is scabies, due to the tiny mite, Acarus scabie.

On 13th July, 1793, he was sitting naked in his bath when a comely young woman from Caen entered. He read the list of names given to him by the girl, Charlotte Corday, then, after sentencing all those on the list to be guillotined, experienced a severe pain in the right upper chest, as the bread knife, brandished by Corday, plunged between the first and second ribs. It transfixed the lung and entered the heart. He cried 'A moi, mon ami!' and died.

Marat belongs among the insane and had the cardinal symptoms of paranoia—intense egoism, delusions of persecution and grandeur. He always considered himself gentle and virtuous, while carrying out deeds of intense brutality and immorality. He had the paranoic's intensity of manner when speaking, utilizing a huge volume of words with which to overwhelm the common man and he always found that the cry 'Les Aristos à la lanterne!' brought him fervent applause from the crowds, the adoration he loved.

And now to another famous French figure. The post mortem examination was carried out on 6th May, 1821: 'The heart, although fatty, was normal. The lungs were also essentially normal, although there were a few adhesions in the pleural cavity and some reddish fluid. The linings of the abdomen were remarkably fat, and the stomach was the seat of extensive disease, many strong adhesions connected to the liver and near the pyloric end an ulcer was found, sufficient to allow passage of the whole of the little finger. The internal surface of the stomach to nearly its whole extent was a mass of cancerous tissue, and contained a large quantity of fluid, resembling coffee grounds. Only the portion near the oesophagus appeared in a healthy state. Apart from the adhesions, the liver presented no unhealthy appearance. The remainder of the abdominal organs were in a healthy state. A slight peculiarity in the formation of the left kidney was observed.'

Thus died Napoleon Bonaparte, from cancer of the stomach developing in the chronic gastric ulcer that had plagued him for so long, causing him to rub his stomach for relief in that classic attitude we shall always associate with him.

In 1756, on a winter's day in January, there was born a son, Wolfgang, to Leopold Mozart, a Bavarian violinist. He had seven children but only this one, and an elder sister, Maria Anna, survived. Wolfgang soon showed outstanding musical ability and by the age of four could play the clavier and tell the pitch of an instrument to the eighth of a tone. At five he started to compose, the score being written down by his father. In 1762 he was taken to Munich to play before Maria Theresa, the Queen of Austria, and then to Vienna to entertain the Imperial Court. During this visit the boy felt increasingly unwell, complaining of a sore throat, fever and pains in the joints and noticed red, painful lumps on his legs and arms. The disease was rheumatic fever.

At the age of eight he began to compose symphonies and sonatas, under the influence of John Christian Bach. In 1767 he developed another infectious disease, smallpox, which left him with deep pock marks on his face, making him very self-conscious (he was also disfigured by a malformed ear which he hid by wearing his hair long).

During the next few years he had recurrent sore throats and joint pains and at twenty-five developed renal colic and an associated infection. The glamour of the early days of the young musical genius had passed and Mozart was poor and in constant ill-health. He worked up to fourteen hours a day, often completely exhausted from fatigue and illness, to pay his ever-pressing creditors.

Mozart became progressively weaker and disillusioned. He had attacks of dizziness, vomiting and headache. His face and body became oedematous and he died on 5th December, 1791, at the age of thirty-four. He was cast into a pauper's grave with nothing to mark the spot.

Throughout life he suffered from recurrent attacks of sore throat and the sequelae rheumatic fever and glomerulonephritis (Bright's disease). It was probably the renal failure that killed him and robbed the world of a true genius who was unappreciated during his lifetime.

In his thirty-seventh year Robert Burns developed a fever, became delirious and died on 21st July, 1796. He had suffered from increasing palpitations of the heart, probably due to mitral stenosis (a disease of the heart due to rheumatic fever), and superadded infection. He had an extraordinary passion for young lassies but there is no medical evidence to support the occasional suggestion that he suffered from venereal disease. In fact he had the same initial disease that killed Mozart, only his heart, not his kidneys, became affected. As he grew older he wrote 'cold, fever and rheumatism have formed to me a terrible combination. I close my eyes in misery and open them without hope.'

Like many original persons, Burns had very little formal schooling and was largely self-educated. Part of his genius was a phenomenal memory; he had a vocabulary of some thirteen thousand words, the same number as Milton, with a Cambridge classical education. He wrote, 'I never had the least thought or inclination of turning poet till I got once heartily in love, and then rhyme and song were the spontaneous language of my heart'.

But in June 1796 he wrote, 'the last three months I have been tortured with an excruciating rheumatism, which has reduced me to the last stave, pale, emaciated and so feeble as occasionally to need help from my chair'. Weak and unable to go upstairs on the 18th July, he collapsed on a kitchen box-bed, where he died three days later from heart failure. His words are forever enshrined in the emotions of his fellow men—'a Man's a Man for a' that'.

Death and misery haunted Edgar Allan Poe, like the spectres and demons from his novels. Born in Boston, Massachusetts in 1809, the second son of a third-rate actor, his mother a beautiful and talented actress, Poe derived all his security and love from her. Miseries and misfortunes plagued him thick and fast. His father died from alcohol, to which he was deeply addicted. His eldest brother died from tuberculosis and his sister, Rosalie, was mentally defective and died in an institution. The shattering blow came when his mother died from tuberculosis at the early age of twenty-four. Poe, profoundly affected, went to live with the family of John Allan, a dour Scottish businessman, who showed the young boy very little affection. At the age of seventeen Poe entered the University of Virginia where he distinguished himself at French and Latin. He now drank considerably and ran into debts which Allan finally refused to pay. He joined the army but his belligerent attitude and refusal to obey orders of his superiors led to a court-martial and dismissal. He began to suffer from recurrent attacks of depression, irritability and despair. At twenty-six Poe married his first cousin, Virginia Clemm. She was thirteen years old. She suffered from constant ill-health and died from tuberculosis at twenty-three. He had very few sexual relations with his wife and suffered from impotence of psychogenic origin and his later sexual relationships were always with women much older than himself, probably as the result of an Oedipus complex.

For many years, in order to overcome his fits of depression, he sought refuge in alcohol and opium. In 1849, having attempted several jobs without success, he was found in a drunken stupor at the polling station in a local election, where he had acted as a 'repeater' (repeated voting was allowed then) and been rewarded with free alcohol. He died from delirium tremens in hospital at the age of forty. Edgar Allan Poe was the victim of manic-depressive psychosis and used alcohol to overcome the depressive crises which occur in the rapid mood swings of this disease. Thus sadly died the originator of the popular *The Murders in the Rue Morgue* and *The Pit and the Pendulum.*

My final famous person was one of the most remarkable, frail, ailing persons of all time. People marvelled that Horatio Nelson was accepted as a midshipman in the harsh rigours of eighteenth-century naval life. But he survived! At the age of sixteen he contracted malaria, while on a visit to the East Indies and it undermined his health to such an extent that he arrived home very weak and emaciated. Later while in the Jamaica Station, he was poisoned by drinking water from a well into which had been thrown branches of the Manchineel apple plant, which contains a poison used by the Indians. He then suffered an acute attack of diarrhoea from typhoid fever which killed 145 of the 200 men. He was very ill for many weeks and at one stage was unable to write because of the nervous weakness due to involvement of the peripheral nerves by the typhoid poison.

In 1784, now a Captain, Nelson developed symptoms of chest pain and the doctors thought he had consumption. He returned to England and spent five years ashore but because he so yearned to go back to sea he eventually persuaded the Admiralty to give him a ship and he returned to the Mediterranean.

While taking part in the siege of Calvi in Corsica a shot struck his battery and a shower of hard splinters hit him in the face, producing detachment of the retina and blindness of the right eye. A few months later the chest pain returned. This was probably an attack of angina due to coronary disease. In 1797, at the Battle of St. Vincent, Nelson was struck on the left side of the abdomen by a cannon ball and this left him with a permanent lump, which may have been a hernia through the torn abdominal muscles. Five months later (July), while attacking Santa Cruz, a musket ball smashed into his right arm, which required immediate amputation.

After an enforced period of rest, he returned to lead the Navy in the Battle of the Nile early in 1798. During this operation he received a severe head wound, resulting in a large flap of skin being separated from the scalp and hanging like a curtain over the left eye. This was replaced on the forehead but although the wound healed quickly he developed headaches and sickness, later to be followed by cough and fever. It was at this time that he was nursed by the notorious Lady Hamilton.

Later, while in Malta, his health deteriorated still further. He suffered from recurrent attacks of gout and abdominal pain, and after the Battle of Copenhagen he became depressed and the pain in his chest returned.

The final outcome is well known. During the Battle of Trafalgar a musket ball penetrated his chest, fracturing part of the shoulder on the left side, smashing the second and third ribs and part of the sixth and seventh thoracic vertebrae. The lungs and main arteries were also severely damaged. He remained composed until death and, although in severe pain, insisted on being kept informed of the progress of the battle. He died assured of one of the greatest naval victories the world has ever seen. It was Nelson who won this battle for Britain and his famous signal at the onset 'England expects ...' typifies the spirit of a man determined to overcome all infirmities and lead by his own inspiration and example.

STRESSES AND STRIFE OF THE MODERN LIFE

IT HAS been said that the treatment of mental disease quite possibly began when the human population of the earth increased from one to two.

The twentieth century has seen the change from the psychoanalytic form of treatment of mental illness to the use of the many chemicals that can affect the mood—the anti-depressants, tranquillizers and sedatives. Psychoanalysis was acknowledged by Freud himself to have definite limitations as a method of treating mental illness. It was considered suitable for the anxiety states, hysteria and obsessional conditions. From the work of Freud, Jung and Adler came such words as introversion, extroversion, the unconscious, ego, id and superego. From the works of Lorenz, Tinbergen and others on mammals and birds has come a complex study of animals' emotions and behavioural instincts. But in animals the feeling of heightened tension humans understand as emotion only occurs when the natural instincts of behaviour are obstructed, in its most excessive state leading to bizarre, undirected and ill-motivated responses. Among lower animals emotion probably plays a very small part, for instincts serve them well within their own environment, from which they rarely stray. But as animals have progressed down the evolutionary scale it has become biologically advantageous to be capable of adaptation to unusual situations. Thus behavioural reflexes have become less rigidly controlled and reasoning and some degree of self-gratification have developed. In man emotion has come to play a greater part in both instinctive and non-instinctive behaviour and he has become adapted for a life that is primarily an accommodation to the conditions and traditions of his own community and civilization. At the same time human beings have been plasticised into a conformity of human development and behaviour, with strong economic and social competitive influences as the motivating forces. Thus conformity to a generally accepted ideal laid down by the community is sought at the expense of individual choices and satisfactions. Many persons are sufficiently plastic to be moulded by their own particular society although they do not all find it equally congenial. The fortunate members adapt and live happily, the unfortunate are ill-adapted and if not supported by the rest of the society there is a gradual decline in ability to cope with external and internal stresses of modern life.

Pavlov approached the understanding of the problems of psychiatry by animal experiments; in his view the life of an animal is a series of adaptations to certain conditioned reflexes acquired throughout its life, new reflexes suppressing old ones in the animal's adaptation to variations in environment. The Pavlovian views, although interesting as basic physiological experiments, are not accepted in their widest sense into modern day psychiatry, although remaining very popular in his native Russia.

In Western society certain modes of action are considered to be normal, this normality really being the average or standard behaviour. If, however, a particular response or trait is exaggerated or inhibited in an individual then he is labelled as suffering from mental illness. The spectrum of normality is broad and often ill-defined and may merge imperceptibly into irrational behaviour. Some mental illnesses so affect the sufferer that the patient's behaviour differs in quality so greatly from the majority that they are easily recognized (the qualitative disorders) whereas others vary in degree (the quantitative disorders).

Of the quantitative disorders, anxiety, depression, irritability, hypochondriasis, paranoid reaction, hysteria and obsession are only variables on the normal individual's response. In the qualitative disorders—schizophrenia, organic brain disease, manic-depressive psychoses and genetic mental deficiencies—there is gross mental aberration. Let us examine some of the commoner mental illnesses and see how they are often only an exaggerated normality experienced by us all.

Now, it is a normal, commonplace experience to be anxious or afraid, fear being an extreme form of reaction to impending danger. However, when the environmental dangers are removed or never existed, then anxiety becomes a quantitative disorder. A tendency towards morbid anxiety is thought to have a genetic or inherited component, but it is also found at the menopause and during the course of several diseases, especially when associated with thyroid overaction. The skin becomes pale and sweating increases, the hands and fingers become restless and fidgety, the lips twitch and the mouth becomes dry. It may be associated with worries (either sexual, financial, social or domestic) a feeling of inferiority in ability and a preoccupation with physical health. Appetite becomes suppressed, swallowing difficult and stomach fullness, nausea and pain related to food are found. Amenorrhoea is common in women, frequency of micturition in men. Sleep is unsatisfying, broken in the early hours and interrupted by vivid dreams and nightmares. Often the sensation of anxiety finally amounts to a feeling of panic.

In depressions the person is characterized by obvious unhappiness, poor concentration, is easily fatigued, suffers loss of energy and libido and has unpleasant dreams and other disturbances of sleep. But, unlike the normal depression we all experience it is out of all proportion to the precipitating circumstances. In its lowest depth there is a real risk of suicide. Usually the depressed state lifts when the unfavourable circumstances alter. There is no daily rhythm in this form of depression, no delusions and almost always some associated causative factor. In manic-depressive psychoses (see later) these phenomena are marked. Apart from the suicide risk, reactive (or circumstantial) depression remits in due course and has a good prognosis.

We all know that certain qualities are found in normal persons and can be regarded as favourable or desirable; these include cleanliness, discipline and orderliness. However, in certain individuals they become developed to a marked degree, and form obsessions and unless they can adhere to strict rules and regulations and follow rigid patterns of behaviour these people become anxious, afraid and insecure. These true obsessional states usually begin insidiously in youth and progress to middle age and later life. The hands must be washed even after touching the cleanest utensils, floors and walls are repeatedly scrubbed (ten, twenty, thirty times per day) to remove infecting organisms, rigid patterns of movement characterize dressing, leaving the office, walking home; taps, doors, switches and gas fittings are checked and rechecked. This ritualistic behaviour may be complicated further by a fear that the ritual has not been satisfactorily carried out and something has been missed and so the whole circle of events begins again. Phobias and imaginary dangers occur, obsessional ruminations run through the mind and may eventually dominate the personality.

In hysteria there is an excessive response to external stresses and it may assume many forms. There may be disturbances of sensation so that pins can be thrust into so-called 'numb' areas of the body. There may be paralysis of the arms or legs and difficulties in walking, especially characterized by ataxia, tremor and a variety of movements. Such 'mental' disturbances were common in troops during both World Wars and often described as a variety of shell shock. Other symptoms include double vision, abdominal pains, menstrual irregularities, alteration in bowel action, skin rashes, and difficulty in breathing and swallowing. In its extreme, the patient passes into a trance-like state and may respond to simple suggestions. Pavlov believed that in hysteria there was a complete breakdown in the nervous integration of the brain and spinal cord. He was able to cause experimental hysteria in animals by training them to react in one way to a stimulus of one variety and in a completely different way to a stimulus which differed from the first only in degree. As the time interval between the two stimuli was brought closer together then the animals had to react in two different manners, until finally, when it was stimulated in two directions at once, hysteria occurred.

In hypochondriasis the person is preoccupied with the whole or one particular region of his body, minutely monitoring each response and sensation seen, felt or experienced in that part. Thus the body image becomes distorted and the person eventually assumes that he is suffering from some organic illness and presents himself in a busy surgery with a logbook of bodily functions extending over the last few months. No amount of reassurance from the doctor helps until he has discussed every point to the last detail; sympathy is often interpreted as signifying that his condition is much worse than he imagined possible, while frank rebuffs are taken as callousness or ignored in his preoccupied perambulations around his own body.

In paranoid reactions there is an abnormal projection and self reference with events, situations and personalities that have in reality only a vague association with the individual concerned. Such traits are common in the sensitive, irritable, touchy, emotionally labile personality. It often springs from lack of self-confidence, feelings of shame and conflicting pride. It is often used as a cover-up for mistakes that would produce some slight loss of esteem in the eyes of friends or fellow workers. Acute paranoid reactions are commoner in the teenager and early adult life than later. In advancing years they may be associated with senility, poor vision and deafness which makes communication with others difficult, and false delusions of persecution, based on fragmentary knowledge, become manifest. Paranoia is seen in schizophrenia in its most bizarre form and under false ideals and impressions acts of a bewildering and sometimes cruel and sadistic nature are carried out, including the murdering of close associates and loved ones.

One of the cardinal features of schizophrenia is that normal persons cannot understand the mental state of the sufferer. The common feature of splitting of the personality is known to everyone, but other disorders of the thought process may be insidious in the early stages of the disease and taken at their face value. In the earliest state consciousness, orientation and memory are not usually affected; perception, sensation and motility may remain undisturbed initially but hallucinations impinge on perception and a peculiar wax-like paralysis on motility. In the simplest form of schizophrenia—incidently a condition that recently occupied almost half of the National Health beds—there is emotional blunting. Since this condition often first occurs in adolescence the young adult is classed as a 'waster', 'drop-out' or 'indifferent, lazy youth'. He (or she) does not care, however, for the rebuffs of his elders. This indifference and callousness may stretch to extremes. Almost always there is a lack of drive and the person drifts casually from job to job, even if one has been acquired in the first place. Schizophrenics slide gently down the social scale (see SLUMS) in blissful serenity. The lack of sensitivity is often present in childhood, although, as I said previously, it becomes more marked in adolescence. Alteration in thought process is not found in the simple cases, but as the condition becomes more marked then lack of concentration, incoherence, wild and irrational mood changes, depression, excitement, tearfulness ensue, finally settling into a permanent state of dreaminess. The expression of emotion in the schizophrenic bears no relation to the ideas expressed —thoughts of death produce sustained laughter, sadness is provoked by a chance, happy remark. The person hears 'voices' which hinder his concentration, command and contradict. Visual disturbances characterized by hallucinations are found. Finally the individual becomes completely absorbed by his 'voices' and listens and converses with them for hours.

In certain other types a negative state is induced, a type of immobile stupor with an associated unresponsiveness to external stimuli such as food, water, questions, commands, etc. In the paranoid states of schizophrenia the persecutory ideas take on a grandiose form.

The causes of schizophrenia are unknown but perhaps genetic factors promote the build-up of toxic chemicals (manufactured by the body and broken down incompletely, or with perhaps defective excretion so they accumulate in the brain) that alter the normal thought processes. In the most severe cases there is a complete breakdown of personality and thought.

Finally, manic-depressive psychosis (like schizophrenia) is a truly qualitative disorder and deserves every ounce of sympathy and understanding. It is characterized by depression of a severe quality, without a recognizable precipitating cause, associated with an elevation of the mood both daily and for indefinite intervals. During the elated periods, self-assertiveness, boastfulness and self-satisfaction are common. There is a flight of ideas, poor association of thoughts and lack of judgement. During the depressive stage there is a complete lack of interest in work and recreation, decisions become difficult, apathy manifest and the person ruminates on thoughts of a morbid or gloomy nature. He or she becomes preoccupied with feelings of guilt and self-reproach, everything that happens to him is interpreted as being due to the fact that he is despised, punished or avoided by his friends and family. Given time, spontaneous remissions are expected but suicide is always a risk. It is often better not to cheer up these persons as the contrast between their own sadness and the happiness of others makes them even more depressed.

The understanding of mental illness is still, in many ways,

in its infancy, although the therapeutic advance in drug treatment has been one of the outstanding medical achievements of the past decade. As the qualitative disorders become suppressed by medical control, the quantitative disorders will become more prominent as the stresses and strains of society mould us in this modern life.

SEX

LIPSTICK, ROUGE, bustles, brassières, bluebottoms, red noses, rich song, elaborate strutting, gorgeous tail-feathers, delicate plumes bright colours—such are the intricate trimmings of sexual selection. The female attracts the male by scent, colour, call or form. The male responds by a direct approach, is easily aroused, tender, loving, lustful, affectionate.

Sex is important in the animal world—only the lowest species reproduce asexually by division. Sex means procreation and procreation means continued survival of the species concerned. Man and the other animals exist in a struggle for survival and a struggle for reproduction. Sexual selection by physical combat, or the threat of combat, characterizes most animals and in the male of the species leads to the development of size and strength necessary for conflict, the formation of weapons of war and devices to make themselves appear larger and more formidable. Thus the tusks of the wild boar, the rich array of antlers in the stag, the manes of lions and bison, the huge jaws of the stage beetle and the large claws of the lobster serve in physical combat, not only to ward off competitors for the female but to disperse the males so that the species is not cramped into small areas but spread evenly throughout the countryside. The rich call of the blackbird at dusk, the red breast of the robin, the breaking of lower tree branches by the roe deer and the deposition of scents by the special anal glands of the civet cat, all serve to mark out territory and warn male trespassers to keep clear and invite females to enter.

In his book, *The Descent of Man and Selection in Relations to Sex* Charles Darwin emphasized the importance of attraction to the male by the female in most creatures, a notable exception being man. In polygamous mammals like the sea elephant the superiority of the males in strength and size is enormous. The inflatable proboscis on the male serves to increase its size. The same occurs in red deer for the most richly endowed antlered male will dominate. Thus the successful males will possess many females, the unsuccessful ones none. Such secondary sex characteristics as the antlers in the male deer are often shed outside the breeding season when their size becomes an encumbrance and a hazard to survival. Their appearance precedes the rutting season and is due to the secretion of hormones by the male sex organs, the testes. Normally in humans the testes descend at birth from the abdomen and lie in the scrotal sac protected from the heat of the body. In many animals they lie within the abdomen and in some, like the deer, they only descend during the mating period.

In birds there is a preponderance of display. The males of most bird species are brightly coloured, the females being smaller and drabber by comparison. The males often have striking colours and patterns restricted to specially developed parts of the plumage (the peacock's tail, the plumes of the bird of paradise) and they indulge in elaborate manoeuvres to show off these bright colours. One variety of bower bird, a drab little brown creature of New Guinea, builds a large structure up to nine feet high of sticks, stones, flowers and leaves and then proceeds to dart round it displaying a gorgeous orange rump, not normally perceived, to the watching female. It is interesting that in this species the bower gets taller the more insignificant the plumage, the missing hues being agumented by the colours of the structure and the bright berries the males carry in their beaks. Even in fish and insects the males will indulge in a variety of subterfuges and combats to gain the affection of the female.

In man, however, the mate selection is usually of women by men and thus the woman deliberately enhances her charms by make-up, fine clothes and a variety of artificial aids. Different races and cultural groups have different standards of beauty and attractiveness. The giraffe-necked women of Burma emphasize the length of their necks by numerous rings applied from childhood while some African tribes insert large discs in the lower lips for attraction. The ultimate aim of all such adornment is reproduction, whether it be man or animal, bird or fish.

From the mutual display techniques of male and female springs the sexual attraction and stimulation. It may be very surreptitious. 'The ceremony of introduction was very soon performed and in two minutes thereafter Mr. Pickwick was joking with the young ladies who wouldn't come over the stile while he looked, or who, having pretty feet and unexceptional ankles, preferred standing on the toprail for five minutes or so and declaring that they were too frightened to move, with as much ease and absence of reserve or constraint, as if he had known them for life. It is worthy of remark too, that Mr. Snodgrass offered Emily far more assistance than the absolute terrors of the stile (although it was full three feet high and had only a couple of stepping stones) would seem to require, while one black-eyed young lady in a very nice little pair of boots with fur round the top was observed to scream very loudly, when Mr. Winkle offered to help her over.' Thus, in his modest way, Dickens described the attraction between male and female in the middle-class, Victorian society. How differently it is handled today.

Sexual behaviour is determined by hormones which are in turn dependent upon the master gland, the conductor of the hormonal orchestra, the pituitary gland. This lies behind the eyes on the base of the brain. In mammals, like sheep and rodents with seasonal breeding, the intensity and duration of light in relation to darkness is transmitted by the retina

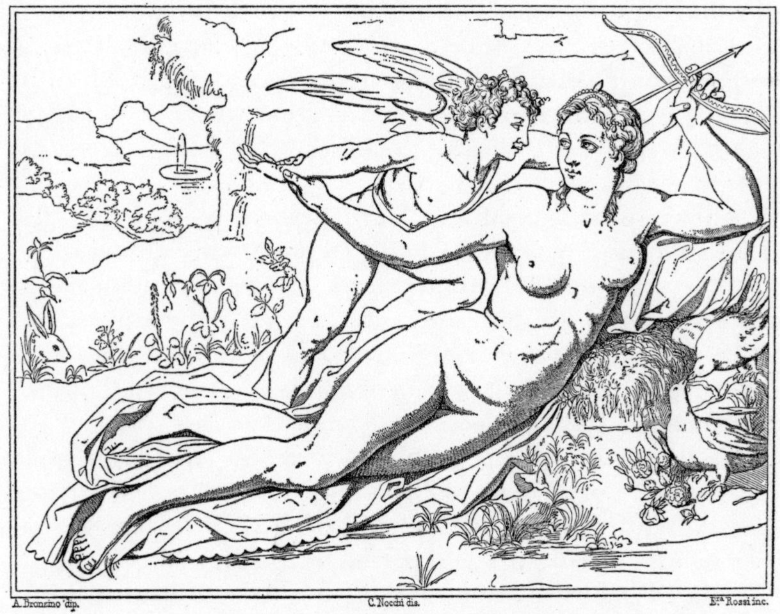

Venus and Cupid. *Rossi after Bronzino*

of the eyes to the brain and the pituitary gland. Once a certain light threshold is reached hormones pour out of the gland and stimulate the ovaries (female) and testes (male) to develop. Once the eggs and sperm reach maturity, secondary sexual attractions and stimulations occur (the secretion of perianal glands, the development of behavioural cries and attitudes) which synchronize maturation and copulation. Since copulation is a relatively unsafe and thus precarious state for the animal, concerned as he must be with predators and survival, it is usually of short duration and effective in fertilization. Only in the human is copulation excessive and unrelated to egg maturation. Most animals at the time of highest sexual activity ovulate and the eggs are released, in a variety of numbers, as the sperm is shed in the genital tract. This phenomenon is very occasionally observed in human females. Another confusing feature of difference between humans and animals is that 'heat' or oestrus in an animal, the period of maximum fertilization, is accompanied by secretion and bleeding, whereas in the human female bleeding usually only occurs during menstruation when the lining of the uterus is shed, due to a fall-off of hormones from the pituitary and ovaries.

The pituitary produces hormones in both sexes. The gradual maturity of this gland, coupled with an increased secretion of gonadotrophins, leads to the development of testes, ovaries, breasts, and other secondary features. This is the period of puberty. The removal of the pituitary from the young animal leaves it physically and sexually retarded, but mentally active, a perpetual Peter Pan.

At the age of twelve or so in the female the signal is received by the ovaries. These pearly-white, walnut-shaped organs, packed with 750,000 tiny ova, begin to shed their eggs, one per month, during the mid-period of the cycle. Each egg has lain in dormant division since it was first produced in the foetus and many will wait for another thirty years or more for their release, most will degenerate with old age and only a few will be fertilized.

The situation in the male is vastly different. Here millions of cells are produced at puberty, each ovoid-shaped testis consisting of six to nine hundred tortuous tubes measuring two foot six inches in length. These pour male cells out and into the long coiled tube of the epididymis beyond. This organ is twenty feet in length and stores the immobile cells in vast numbers. They will survive for a short period—a few days at 4°C but a few years at -79°C. Each ejaculation contains over five hundred million live, wriggling, tadpole-like spermatozoa, enough to fertilize each woman of reproductive age in the world. During copulation these cells, still immobile, are shunted past and admixed with the secretions of the prostate gland and seminal vesicles. These secretions protect, vivify and nourish the sperm in the female genital tract. Each spermatozon measures 45μ: the length of the reproductive apparatus in the female, from the upper vagina to the ampulla of the uterine tube where fertilization takes place is 7·8 inches. The journey of the sperm corresponds to a man traversing 5·05 miles. But Nature is prepared.

Before coitus the penis becomes erect due to the engorgement of its blood vessels brought about chiefly by the dilatation of the arteries and the contraction of small muscles that obstruct the venous outflow from the organ. In a woman the clitoris also becomes erect and the vulva and vagina secrete mucous fluid which facilitates the passage of the penis in the vagina. Coitus, which usually lasts for only a few minutes, culminates in the orgasm, during which the semen is ejaculated by rhythmic contractions of the perineal muscles. During orgasm in the female, which should occur at the same time, the neck to the womb dilates and spermatozoa pass through. (It has been shown that sperm are found in the uterine tube of the cow after only two and a half minutes, having travelled twenty inches in that time.) Coitus is a reflex action through the lower part of the spinal cord and damage to that region in the male may prevent it from occurring, but it is accompanied by psychic excitement and must be regarded as a cerebral event.

The race is now on. Out of the 500-million cells only one is needed for fertilization in most instances. But pregnancy does not occur unless these vast numbers are deposited. It is thought that it is necessary to have such a large number to supply sufficient enzymes to dissolve the jelly-like lining of the outer case of the egg, but this has been doubted by some observers. Freshly ejaculated spermatozoa do not appear to be able to enter the ovum. They acquire this capacity after a few hours stay in the reproductive tract. Fertilization takes place within twelve hours of coitus in man, the spermatozoa only surviving about twenty-four hours. This is due to the relatively high temperature of the vagina and uterus as compared to the scrotum. In the rabbit they survive four days and ovulation occurs twelve hours after mating. If the doe rabbit is mated with a sterile buck then pseudo-pregnancy is produced for a short period. In the rabbit the maximum life of the ovum is six hours, in the guinea pig thirty-two hours and in the human eighteen to twenty-four hours. Ovulation in man usually takes place on the 12-15 day of the cycle but can be found over a wide range (6-20 days). It is claimed that there is a slight fall of body temperature followed by a slight rise of 0·5 °C, in the middle of the menstrual cycle that indicates the time of ovulation. Unfortunately, this change in temperature may follow two to three days later in some cases. The mucus secreted by the cervix has certain properties which can be detected by chemical means at the time of maximum fertilization and has been used as a test for ovulation.

Once the spermatozoan *has* penetrated the ovum the rest are repelled. Now the egg begins to divide, at first forming a conglomeration of cells, that change into a ball-like shape, meanwhile being borne on the delicate, hair-like processes of the cells that line the uterine tube back to the body of the uterus.

This return to the womb is vital. Should it be arrested by disease then the fertilized egg will die but it may attempt to survive in this foreign situation. If the nourishment is sufficient here it can develop into a normal baby to be delivered by operation. However, it usually perishes. Sometimes it erodes through the tubal wall and into the abdominal cavity—a ruptured ectopic pregnancy. Very, very rarely such a foetus may grow in the abdomen, obtaining nourishment from the lining of the bowel walls and a few cases have been recorded of a living child being found at operation. Often they are converted into stone, miniature calcium effigies of a normal human being and recently a thirty-seven-year-old child was removed from a seventy-four-year-old woman, the child being completely converted into stone. Similar monstrosities have been found in Egyptian mummies.

The next crucial stage is the burrowing of the fertilized

ovum into the special, spongy, highly vascular wall of the womb. Like a tiny mite it burrows on the sixth to eighth day after conception, obtaining nourishment from its own 'yolk' cells, and the tissues it engulfs. During this period a mass of cells become highly specialized and produce a hormone similar to the one mentioned in the pituitary—called chorionic gonadotrophin. This substance is carried by the blood stream back to the ovary and maintains the residual husk of the egg follicle, still on the surface of the gland, from which the ovum originally ruptured. This remaining structure is called the corpus luteum (or yellow body) because of the colour of its cells. They are important producers of progesterone, one of the female hormones, that keeps the uterus in a state of preparation prior to fertilization; should fertilization not be successful then the level of progesterone falls and the lining of the uterus sheds as menstrual fluid. The chorionic gonadotrophin signals to the corpus luteum to continue progesterone production and also initiates the outpouring of another female hormone called oestrogen. Later the placenta takes over the production of chorionic gonadotrophin. Incidentally it is this hormone that has been so long used in various pregnancy tests. After three weeks the level rises and can be detected in the urine. If injected into the South African clawed toad, Xenopus, it lays eggs within twenty-four hours. Other animal tests involving rabbits and mice used to be used but are now supplanted by direct chemical/immunological methods in the laboratory, giving accurate results within minutes.

The foetus now begins to develop and from a single cell, in only nine months, a baby will be constructed, with a variety of tissues, functionally perfect.

Muller once remarked 'ontogeny recapitulates phylogeny' the development of the egg recreates the evolution of the organism. From the single cell comes an amoeba-like creature, then a ball of cells, through the double cell layer, then the three cell layer, with the development of the heart as primitive as any reptile, the brain as small as any crustacean, then with fish-like gills, that only persist as the small bones in the throat (Adam's apple and hyoid bone above) and the mandible, through the ape-like stage of dense hair covering, to the final human form. Evolution that took five hundred million years re-enacted in nine months!

Half the baby's weight is acquired during the last six weeks of pregnancy. During the first two weeks the egg becomes purely a mass of cells, and measures $\frac{1}{4}''$ (6 mm.). Between two and four weeks the head and tail folds develop (4·2 mm. or $\frac{1}{6}''$, because of folding) and the primitive organs and vessels are seen. The primitive circulation begins. In the fifth week the embryo becomes markedly curved like a letter C, the yolk sac becomes more definitely pinched off and connected through a narrow duct, the gill arches appear and the rudiments of the eyes, ears and limb buds can be identified. By the seventh week (15 mm. or $\frac{1}{2}''$) the head and brain are more conspicuous, and the acute curvature starts to straighten out. The limbs elongate, the liver and heart are prominent and the bowel lies formed outside the abdominal cavity which is filled with the liver, urinary and reproductive organs. The external genitalia appear and the tail begins to disappear. The eyelids become separated from the eye. By the eighth week (1″ or 25 mm.) almost all the organs have been formed and the fingers and toes appear. In the third month the head is extended and the neck lengthened, the eyelids meet and fuse, remaining closed until the sixth month, although sight is not fully established until two to three weeks after birth. The limbs are well developed and nails appear on the digits. The bowel coils itself into the rapidly expanding abdominal cavity and the umbilical hernia disappears. The foetus now measures 10 mm. ($4\frac{1}{2}''$). In the fourth month lanugo (or fine hair) appears on the body and the total length is now 14 cm. ($5\frac{3}{4}''$) body, with legs extended 22 cm. ($8\frac{1}{2}''$). During the fifth month the foetus starts to move and hair begins to grow on the head. The total length becomes 30 cm. (12″). The skin becomes greasy. By twenty-four weeks the length is 33 cm. and weight is 2½ lbs. (1 kilo). In the seventh month the eyelids open, the testes descend to the groin and the skin is red and wrinkled, giving the appearance of an old man. The weight is 1·5 kilo (3½ lbs.) and size 40 cm. (16″). In the eighth month the fine hair vanishes and the fat is deposited in the skin to give the characteristic chubby look (now 45 cm., 2·5 kilo). In the ninth month the testes enter the scrotum, the length of the child is 20″ and the weight is 7 lbs. In animals the size of the baby is determined by the size of the mother. If, as in Walton and Hammond's classical artificial insemination experiment, a shire mare is crossed with a shetland stallion and vice versa, the shetland mare had a small foal, while the other was almost of normal size for the mother. These factors are not so important in the human. The smallest recorded birth weight and survival is 10 oz., the largest 24 lbs. 4 oz. During pregnancy the hormone levels in the blood rise. The oestrogens prepare the breasts, causing them to enlarge and the milk cells to multiply, and they also produce the initial nausea and the dilation of blood vessels, noticeable as varicose veins. The progesterones relax the muscles of the uterus, which enlarge tenfold, and the ligaments of the pelvis, giving the pregnant women a peculiar waddling gait and also backache. After delivery these hormones rapidly decrease to normal levels, the pituitary then releases another hormone (prolactin) to cause milk secretion. Should milk production be excessive, or have to be controlled on medical grounds, then oestrogens are prescribed to stop the pituitary from secreting prolactin. This procedure is familiar to thousands of women who have had lactation problems.

Finally, the above hormones, oestrogen and progesterone, have been combined to produce a state of mini-pregnancy, as a means of contraception. This is the pill. First conceived by Pincus in 1956, who had observed that rabbits did not ovulate when given progesterone, and then found that contraception occurred when women were given 300 mg. of progesterone by mouth from the fifth to the twenty-fifth day of the cycle. Since then many synthetic hormonal substances have been manufactured and the first large scale trial was carried out in Puerto Rico. This was a success and 'the pill' found to be one hundred per cent effective if taken properly, with a return to normal fertility immediately after stopping the tablets.

The pill acts by dampening down the pituitary hormones, stopping ovulation and increasing the stickiness of the mucus at the neck of the womb so that the spermatozoa cannot pass through. Some of the more recent pills have been aimed at only the latter effect but have a higher than average failure rate. The short term dangers of the pill are well known. The oestrogen can affect the clotting mechanism of the blood, producing thrombosis and embolism. But this is a rare event. In a recent survey the chances of pulmonary embolus occurring through use of the pill was found to be 3 in 100,000 women, the chance of embolism of pregnancy was 9 per 100,000. It is probably the oestrogen content (that has recently been reduced by the Warning Committee on Drug Safety) that alters the level of various fatty components and platelets in the blood, thus linking the use of the drugs with thrombosis. However, the pill is effective, the failure rate being less than 1 per 100 women years. With other methods of contraception corresponding figures are I.U.D. (intra-uterine device) less than 5, diaphragm 12, safe period 14, condom 15, douche 15, coitus interruptus 16, local spermicides 21. Thus it has been computed that of a million people on the pill less than 23 would die from its effects. whereas approximately 51 would die from the associated pregnancy from the failure of these other methods. At present there is no need for undue alarm about 'the pill', providing its use is controlled by the family doctor and no doubt it will remain in the forefront of great medical advances of the twentieth century.

THE PROUD SHEPHERD, SYPHILIS

A shepherd once (distrust not ancient fame)
Possest these downs, and Syphilis his name.
A thousand heifers in these vales he fed,
A thousand ewes to those fair rivers led.

THUS WROTE Hieronymus Fracastorius, the famous Italian physician, in his epic poem, *A Poetical History of the French Disease*. The poem, although written in a light-hearted manner, became so famous that the word syphilis is now the universal term for this disease. The poem relates the legend of the shepherd, Syphilis, who, for an act of unfaithfulness, namely the erection of an altar to the god, Alcithous, was smitten by the 'all-seeing Sun'. He—

First wore Buboes dreadful to the sight,
First felt strange pains and sleepless past the night.
From him the malady received its name,
The neighbouring Shepherd catcht the spreading Flame.

The origin of syphilis, the 'spreading flame' is shrouded in mystery. The theory that syphilis was introduced into Europe by the sailors of Columbus has been accepted for many years. These sailors had, according to legend, contracted the disease from the natives of America. The first general outbreak was in Naples in 1495 amongst the troops in the army of Charles, and by the end of the fifteenth and early sixteenth century this disease was beginning to attract great attention. In 1498

Leoniceno wrote a small treatise called *The French Disease*, stating that the malady was known to Hippocrates and other ancient physicians, and noting 'The French disease has pustules at first on the private, then the rest of the body and commonly accompanied with great pain'. He did not stress the importance of sexual contact, although he recognized the extreme contagiousness of the disease.

Villabos (1498), the Spanish physician, referred to the early appearance of a small ulcer on the external genitalia before the generalized spread. 'Thus 'tis the passion on these members is presented many days before it yet hath appeared in other places.'

But it was the careful study of Johannis de Vigo (1460-1520), surgeon to Pope Julius II, which stressed the origin of syphilis from sexual intercourse with an infected person. 'Thys dysease is contagious, chiefly yf it chaunce through copulation of a man wyth an unclene woman, for the begynnygne therof was in the secret members of men and women, with lytle pushes of vlewe colour, otherwhyles of blacke, sometyme of whytyshe, wyth a certayn hardness aboute the same.' Thus he described quite accurately the early primary lesion, (the indurated chancre), and goes on to talk about the secondary rashes and ulcers and the final gummata (or large necrotic lumps in the internal organs and skin).

Jacques de Bethencourt, the French physician, rejected the term 'French disease' and suggested since the disease arises from illicit love it 'should be called the malady of Venus, or venereal disease'. He wrote 'the venereal disease is a condition of the body from sexual intercourse and contagion: at the onset causing ulcers on the genitalia or the point of contagion: then corrupting the humors, especially the phlegm, the organs of generation: by which pustules, tumors, ulcers and pains are produced'.

During the eighteenth century one doctor towered above all others, his name John Hunter, the greatest name in the history of British surgery. Amongst his many thousands of experiments he came to the conclusion that gonorrhoea and syphilis were the same disease, and carried out a hazardous experiment on himself (1767). 'Two punctures were made on the penis with a lancet dipped in venereal matter from a gonorrhoea; one puncture was on the glans, the other on the prepuce.' Hunter rapidly developed syphilis and in 1773, six years later, was very ill with a large aneurysmal swelling of the main artery of the chest, the aorta. During a heated argument he 'went into the next room and turning to a friend, gave a deep groan and dropt down dead'. His aneurysm had ruptured.

The diagnosis of syphilis was revolutionized by the discovery in 1905, by Schaudinn, a Prussian zoologist, of the causative organism Treponema pallidum. It is a spiral-shaped structure, resembling a corkscrew, with eight spirals and measures 8μ in length. The incubation period of syphilis is from ten to ninety days. In ninety-six per cent of the cases, the primary sore or chancre is situated on the genital organs. In the male it is usually obvious but in the female the primary sore on the inner aspect of the vulva or cervix of the womb is often unnoticed by the patient, and the infection is likely to progress well into the second stage before its true nature is recognized. But these sores can be found on other regions of the body. This point is often unappreciated by the general public. They have been found on the lips (mainly on the upper), the nipples and fingers. Primary sores of the lips and mouth usually result from kissing and it has been recorded that five young ladies were infected by one young man at a dance. Indiscriminate kissers beware! Dentists and obstetricians are prone to inoculation on the fingers.

The primary lesion presents as a thickened lump, which becomes oedematous and ulcerates. In many cases more than one chancre appears. After healing the secondary stage takes between two and twelve months to appear. The general features include anaemia, malaise, lymph node enlargement, rashes and ulcers and warts in the mouth and genital region.

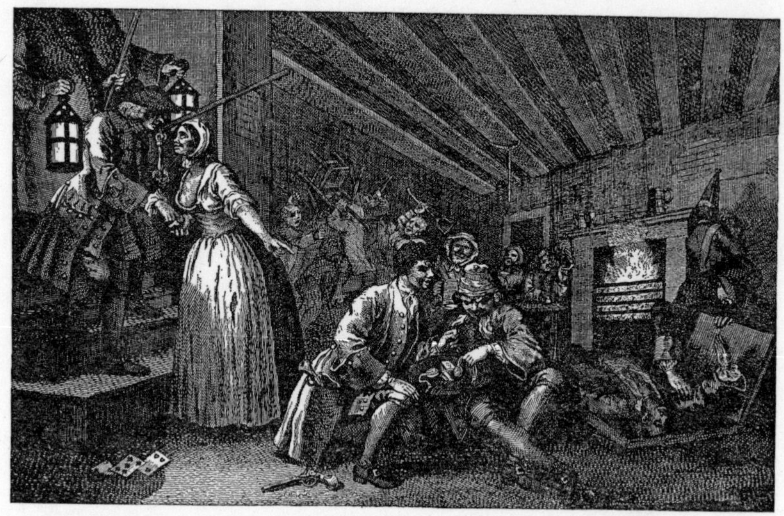

The Idle Prentice betrayed by his Whore and taken in a Night Cellar. *Hogarth*

At a late period of the second stage, fleeting bone pains, testicular pain and swelling and eye inflammation ensue.

In the third and final stage, commencing three years after the initial lesion, large fibrous, necrotic gumma appear, that break down on the skin and form a sloughing ulcer. Gumma may be found in internal organs, chiefly the liver. They are nearly always painless, although bone erosion becomes painful. If they heal on the skin they leave a thin 'tissue-paper scar'. Finally, changes occur in the nerves to the legs producing unco-ordinated walking, and in the cells of the brain leading to general paralysis of the insane. This constitutes a gross alteration in behaviour, grandiose ideas, loss of memory and ultimate dementia. Destruction of other organs can occur at any stage. The joints especially the knees, and the large blood vessels are particularly affected. Ruptured aortic aneurysms were once the primary killers of young men with syphilis and still occasionally occur.

But the greatest inherent danger of syphilis is its effect on the developing foetus. Many abort, or are stillborn. Those that survive have all the features of congenital syphilis—patchy hair, blindness, poor vision, ear trouble, joint deformity and a characteristic face (the halt, the blind, the deaf and the impotent).

The treatment of syphilis was unknown until 1909 when Paul Ehrlich, at his 606th attempt, produced an arsenic compound, Salvarsan. Bismuth injections were then found to be effective. However, after the discovery of penicillin an effective total cure was instituted by a course of injections. But syphilis is still not eradicated and during the last decade there has been an alarming increase in the number of new venereal disease cases reported, especially in young people.

If syphilis is not diagnosed early (and many people are still ignorant of the presenting symptoms of the disease) then it can cause great ill-health and an increasing mortality. Despite the advent of antibiotics, the proud Shepherd still reigns, and 'neighbours catch the spreading flame'.

CORONARY THROMBOSIS

MODERN MAN has other problems, however, one of the most urgent being coronary thrombosis that kills in the prime of life. Often the unfortunate victim is a young man in his thirties, with a young wife and family. A sudden tight chest pain, a breathless collapse, with ashen face, distended veins and perspiration on the temples and another statistic is filed away on the forms of the Registrar General.

What can be done to prevent it? What is the problem? In simple anatomical terms the arteries to the heart are end-arteries, that is to say that they, and they alone, can supply a given sector of the cardiac muscle. Once blocked, the blood containing oxygen and other nourishing substances cannot reach the ischaemic area to feed the muscle fibres and the heart begins to fail—or go into uncontrollable fluttering action (correctly called fibrillation), when the fibres contract asymetrically and in an unco-ordinated manner. Such are the remarkable reserves of the heart that it can often maintain the blood pressure and circulation and the patient will survive. Sometimes he succumbs either from massive cardiac damage or simple fibrillation. In the latter instance a recovery may be facilitated in a hospital by the application of a defibrillating machine which shoots a high voltage electric current through the chest, thus completely stopping all activity in the heart. Now external pressure, rhythmically to the chest wall, can pump the blood around the vessels in the body and the heart may start beating again. Such external cardiac massage, coupled with mouth to mouth respiration, has resulted in the saving of thousands of lives following a heart attack. This technique should never be applied to the living (e.g. a simple faint) by an inexperienced person. First aid centres run courses in instruction.

But to return to the original problems.

In the field of preventive medicine there are still many questions to answer. The root cause of the trouble is small, fatty plaques (called atheroma) that develop in the arteries in the body. How do they get there?

The normal pressure in our arteries at rest is at least 120 m.m. of mercury and any factor that promotes eddy currents, for example, at the bifurcation of two vessels, produces stresses in the delicate lining of the artery wall. Then fatty material, usually derived from ingested cholesterol and other animal fats, is deposited at these sites and eventually builds into small streaks and later plaques that can either obstruct the blood flow or form small clots of blood (since blood will adhere to any roughened surface) which is called thrombosis. One of these clots can grow until it occludes the lumen of the artery, or break off and embolise down the vessel in the direction of flow. Like debris caught in a stream it is eventually trapped, causing stagnation and further clotting behind it. The effects produced depend upon the size of the vessel blocked and whether blood can reach the cells concerned by using another route. If not, these ischaemic cells perish and an area of dead tissue remains (called an infarct). This tissue is eventually digested by white corpuscles and replaced with dense fibrous material, the binding component of the body.

One logical method to reduce the incidence of coronary thrombosis is to decrease the intake of animal fats e.g. butter, cream, lards etc. But this is not the complete answer, for herbivores in the wild state can also develop fatty streaks (atheroma) which must be of little comfort if you are a rhinoceros or an eland deer. Whether they later go on to form coronary thrombosis is another matter, and most scientists think not.

Exercise is important. This does not mean suddenly leaping out of a chair and dashing down the street at fifteen miles an hour or setting off on a ten mile hike. It means an increase in exercising capabilities over a period of months to reach a steady state for performance and then maintaining that degree of exercise. People who exercise regularly have, in general, a decreased chance of having a heart attack, exercise promoting blood flow and reducing body fat. Being slim is very important!

Finally, being a woman certainly helps, because the incidence of this condition in females is greatly lower than in males. This fact is thought to be due to the fat-clearing effect of the female hormone, oestrogen, on the blood. There is no question, however, of a woman's femininity being assessed by whether she has a coronary thrombosis or not.

Surgery is at present almost useless in this disease. Some surgeons have attempted to core out the diseased fatty material in a reboring operation; others have transplanted vascular areas from different regions in order to improve the blood supply, but both procedures have had little success. Perhaps in years to come preventive medicine will provide the answer but at the moment it deserves all the attention that science is devoting to it.

SPORT AND EXERCISE AS THE KEY TO PHYSICAL FITNESS

LONG BEFORE the first Olympic games were staged at Olympia in 776 B.C. the Greek people had developed a taste for sports that elevated athletic games to a prominent place in their daily lives. Sports competitions among the Greeks began with a religious orientation, for contests of physical strength and skill were believed to invigorate and renew the youth of the participants, to achieve the powers of the gods and restore to the dead, living as a pale reflection of life in the earth, some hidden powers. Funeral ceremonies and athletic tournaments often went hand in hand. Generally sport became cultivated for its health-giving properties only, and as a preparation for, or peaceful alternative to, combat. In order to develop their ideals of perfection and beauty in both body and mind, sport became an essential part of the school curriculum. Homer describes horse-racing, boxing, wrestling, foot-races, archery and combat with weapons, but many of the techniques in these well-known sports were widely different from today. The boxers used oxhide bindings to cover their fists and aimed all the blows at the opponent's head and face, which explains why the ancient fighters, unlike boxers of today, always seemed to have their arms raised. The combat went on without interruption until one of the boxers was totally unable to continue, his face often badly cut and bruised from the oxhide strips. 'With one mighty blow I will tear his flesh to ribbons' was the cry of Epeius, a Greek boxing champion. Wrestling was the most popular sport in Ancient Greece, a combat of strength, balance, swiftness, skill and judgement. Victory went to the man who felled his opponent three times. Discus-throwing utilized an underhand throw, the javelin was hurled with the aid of a leather thong passed round the shaft and on to the second and third finger of the athlete, while the long jumper held weights in each hand to gain momentum and to keep himself from falling back at the end of the jump. The participating athletes, freeborn Greeks, went into intensive training for a month beforehand. The Olympic Games lasted until A.D. 393, a period of nearly twelve centuries. Finally denigrated by the Romans to barbaric events and circuses, the Games were to vanish until 1896 when the first modern Olympic Games was held in Athens. Meanwhile, cruel Norsemen had played a game which consisted of kicking a human skull or head belonging to an enemy; English peasants had grappled and kicked pigs' bladders filled with air between two landmarks many miles apart; the Tudor and Scottish kings had played at Royal Tennis, while golf began to appear among the populace of the north of Britain. But it was not until the nineteenth century, with its overcrowding, and industrial expansion that sport began to be organized in a great way and the modern cults of soccer, rugger, cricket, golf and athletics became truly established.

But what effects does athletic exercise have on the human body? Anyone who participates in a sport after a long lay-off or sedentary occupation appreciates the difference between occupational and athletic fitness. This has led to often asserted dogma that exercise is for the young, that the so-called 'aged' of thirty-five-plus years should content themselves with a gentle game of golf, a swim in the summer and a game of chess. At all periods of life sport and exercise is beneficial. It is true that professional athletes who train to extremes may

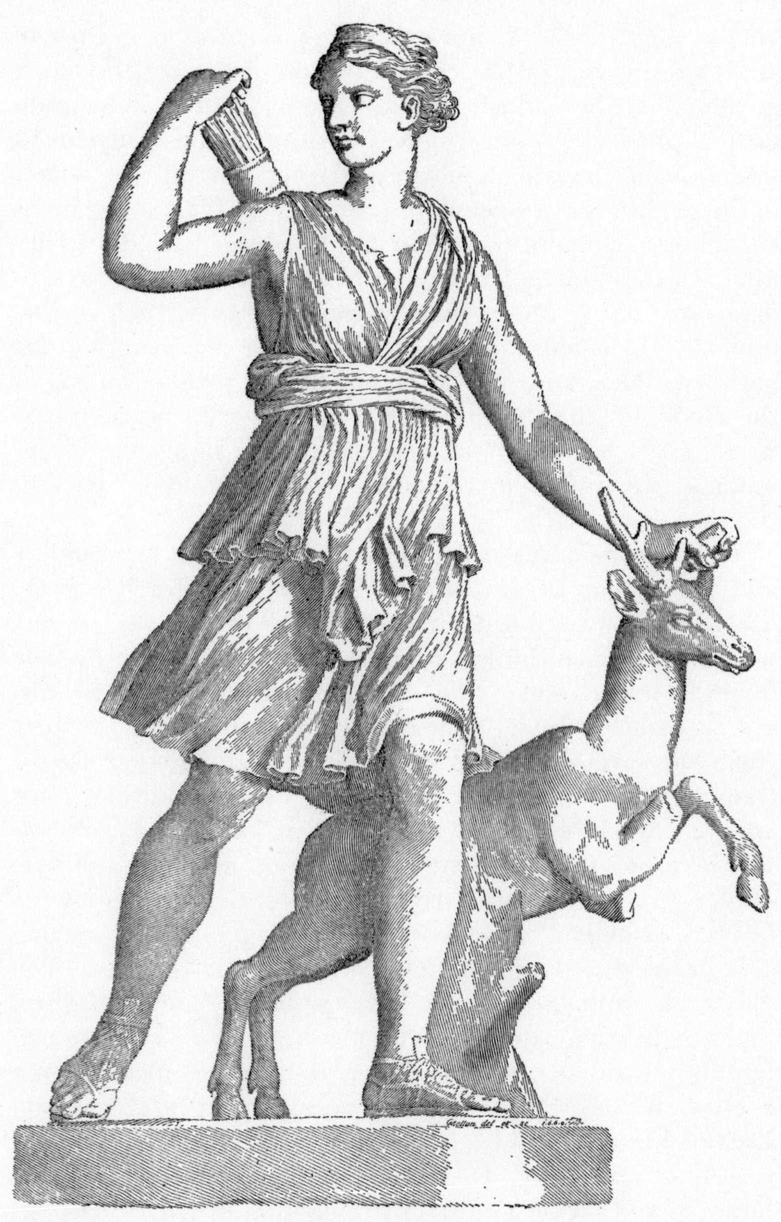

Diana. *Mellan*

have a slightly shorter life expectancy but this is not necessarily proven and in fact their duration of life will be much greater than the paunchy, middle-aged executive, having no greater physical stresses imposed on him than a casual stroll to the car or elevating a leisurely glass of martini. The secret to physical fitness is to explore it gradually. Walk a few miles daily before attempting to insert a few brief periods of running. Do a few light exercises and draw a few deep breaths before partaking in any mild exercise. Increase each regime gradually to avoid sudden stresses on the ligaments of the back, shoulder, knee and ankle, or pulled muscles chiefly at the elbow or knee. Exercise is associated with an increased strength of contraction in muscles, power in ligaments and tendons, movement in joints and alteration in capacity of the lungs and heart.

Each year an adult human inhales and exhales beween two and five million litres of air, twenty per cent of which is O_2. These gases swirl down the passageways to the tiny air sacs where the oxygen diffuses into the blood and carbon dioxide leaves it. In the human lung the surface area available for this gas exchange is huge, some seventy square metres, or forty times the surface of the adult body. Accordingly gas can be transferred to and from the blood quickly and in huge amounts. Each breath consists of half a litre of air, each person breathes ten to fourteen times per minute to supply oxygen to the three hundred million alveolar air sacs for the billions of cells of the body that need it. But the carbon dioxide produced by the lungs must also be removed. The maximum human capacity for ventilation is about thirty times the resting rate, a flow of one hundred and fifty to two hundred litres per minute. Even during the most intense exercise, however, the ventilation averages only beween eighty and one hundred and twenty litres a minute—man has a great reserve of ventilation. Of the five hundred mls. per breath, a hundred and fifty are wasted by remaining in the air passages leading to the alveolar air sacs and this is called 'dead space gas'. Because gases flow from regions of higher pressure to lower pressure the air is rapidly distributed amongst the three hundred million sacs, a remarkable feat of natural engineering. During the act of breathing the lungs passively follow the inspiratory expansion of the chest wall (ribs, muscles, etc.) and diaphragm (which separates the chest from the abdomen and moves down towards the abdomen during inspiration) because the pleura (a fine, enclosed cavity of connective tissue which embraces each lung with one surface and the inner side of the chest wall and diaphragm with the other) has a negative pressure within it. If air enters, from a puncture wound for example, into this pleural cavity, then the lung remains collapsed and does not follow the chest movements and respiration is therefore impaired. With the expansion of each lung the pressure of the gas in the alveolar sacs drops and air is sucked in through the nose, mouth, and air passages—a passive phenomenon. The oxygen then diffuses across the very thin alveolar wall and into the capillaries beyond where it is taken up by the haemoglobin of the red blood cells. The length of the capillaries measures several hundreds of miles, but at any one instance contains only 70-100 ml. which is the volume of blood ejected by one heart beat. If the blood did not contain red cells which avidly take up oxygen, then 83 L. of blood would have to pass through the lungs at rest to maintain the oxygen requirements of the body. At high altitudes the pressure of O_2 in the alveolar air sacs falls and the athlete's performance for distance events is poor by comparison with that at sea level. Oxygen is needed to burn glucose in the muscles to produce energy, but a small quantity of glucose can be used without O_2 (anaerobic metabolism). During a sprint race (100 to 220 metres) the athlete obtains all his energy by burning glucose without oxygen. In the 100 metres, for example, he does not take a breath. Up to four hundred metres the energy requirement is met by this anaerobic mechanism and the runner builds up an oxygen debt which he looses at the end of the activity. Thus at high altitudes, where the air is thinner and imparts less friction to the athlete to impede progress, anaerobic events, (e.g. 100-400 metres, long jumping etc.) are characterized by increased performances, as in the Mexico Olympic Games where all these records were broken. Also athletes training at high levels, to combat the low O_2 pressures develop certain metabolic and physiological changes in the body, chiefly an increase in the number of red blood cells, which give him/her an advantage in performance, even when running at sea level. Thus countries like Kenya are now producing athletes of world class ability.

However, the upper limits of exercise depend not upon the lungs, where there is a fantastic reserve in oxygen intake capacity, but upon the heart. It is now established that in a young man the heart can increase its output from 5·5 L. of blood per minute at rest to nearly five times that figure during maximum exertion (25-30 L.). Each heartbeat at rest ejects some 70 ml. of blood, but to obtain the above quantities would require a pulse rate of 360 plus per minute. The normal pulse rate is 70-80 per minute (lower in athletes, i.e. 40-60), and above 180 the heart beats so quickly that it cannot adequately fill with blood and the amount ejected becomes less and less. Thus, some other mechanisms come into play. The heart, after dispensing with the 70 mls. (stroke volume, mentioned above) still contains residual blood of up to 50 mls. or so. During exercise the body utilizes this residual blood and the volume of each stroke of the heart rises to 100-140 mls. or more, with a pulse rate of 120-160 plus. Training improves the muscles of the heart, producing an increase in stroke volume, so that the pulse rate need not rise as quickly as in the untrained and falls to normal within three or so minutes of exercise; it also improves the ventilation and diffusion of oxygen.

The muscles, ligaments and tendons improve in power and extensibility during exercise. Muscle consists of two basic types of fibres, red and white. The white contracts rapidly (e.g. wing muscles of birds attached to 'breast' region) while the red is necessary for sustained muscle contraction (leg muscles in birds). The 'red' colour is due to myoglobin, a substance that is very similar chemically to haemoglobin and incorporates and stabilizes O_2 within the cell in a similar manner to haemoglobin. Animals which require a high level of O_2 in the tissues (diving animals like seals and whales) have a preponderance of myoglobin in their muscles, giving them an almost black appearance. Sprinting and distance running develop the white muscle and static exercises develop the red. For good athletic performance a training regime should be employed that incorporates both running, walking and body-building exercises. In weight-lifting for sports the maximum single-lift weight should be ascertained and reduced by ten to twenty pounds for repeated exercises. Muscles contract in groups and while one group contracts, the muscles on the opposite side of the joint have to relax, or stalemate exists. This co-ordinated action requires complex nervous reflex pathways in the brain and spinal cord. The attainment of skill is the full development of these reflexes. Practice makes skill. Muscles can be damaged by unco-ordinated action. These are the muscle-pull injuries and take place within the main muscle belly, or at its junction with tendons or ligaments. Tendons are composed of collagen (a type of connective tissue) that is enormously strong—in the Achilles tendon during running it supports half a ton per square inch—and often the tendon is torn out of its insertion into bone before it actually ruptures. Ligaments are likewise composed of collagen and stretch, or partially tear, rather than rupture. When completely torn ligaments and tendons require hospital suturing they never regain one hundred per cent strength, seventy per cent being the usual figure.

Exercises bring into play the co-ordinated actions of complex physiological animal systems that have evolved over millions of years and have been allowed to degenerate through misuse and sedentary occupations prevalent in the twentieth century. One is never too old to embark on activity providing it is gradual and does not produce pain. The benefits to health and mental well-being are enormous. Exercise is the key to physical fitness.

ALCOHOL

WHEN ASKED to take a little wine Samuel Johnson replied, 'I can't drink a little, therefore I never touch it.' When he was on Skye Lady McLeod, hardly crediting his reason for refusing to drink, said, 'I am sure, sir, you would not carry it too far,' to which Johnson replied, 'Nay, Madam, it carried me. I took the opportunity of a long illness to leave it off, and having broken off the habit, I have never returned to it.'

Johnson at one stage belonged to the group of pathological drinkers, and like so many of them was amazingly secretive in this respect. 'When I drank wine, I scorned to drink when in company. I have drunk many a bottle by myself; in the first place I needed it to raise my spirits, in the second place, because I would have nobody witness its effects upon me.'

He later remarked reflectively, 'This is one of the disadvantages of wine, it makes a man mistake words for thoughts.' But during the nineteenth and early twentieth centuries the purge against alcohol and gin cellars was at its height. Sir Andrew Clark, Physician to Queen Victoria said, 'Alcohol is a poison—so is strychnine, so is arsenic. It ranks with these agents. More than three-fourths of the disorders in what we call "fashionable life" arise from the use of alcohol.' While Sir Edward Fry (1905), the Lord Justice of Appeal, noting the steady rise of alcoholic 'insanity', cried, 'The vast increase of lunatics in this country demands the serious consideration of every means to protect society from physical and mental degeneration.' 'It is most sad and discouraging that this preventable cause of the most terrible of all human diseases should thus continue to increase. It is a veritable plague spot in our social life.' (Clouston 1903.)

'If I could destroy tomorrow the desire for strong drink in the people of Britain,' thundered Joseph Chamberlain in 1874, 'what changes we should see. We should see our gaols and workhouses empty.'

Alcohol had been considered as a food, sedative and anaesthetic for many generations up to this time. Prior to the 1840's when anaesthesia had been developed, amputations were often performed swiftly under alcoholic stupor. But the dangers of these beverages on the stomach were sounded most emphatically.

Mease (1831) in the treatment of sick-headaches due to upset gastric function, advocates that 'the tonic effect of malt liquors are injurious and, therefore, must be avoided'. The best solvent for our food is *pure water.* Recalling that 'every man is his own physician at forty years of age' he prescribes a light diet—wild meats being more tender than domestic animals, must be eaten whenever possible, an abundance of venison is most proper. Game of all kinds and rabbits, beef, good mutton, beeve's tongues (properly salted and smoked) and corned beef are proper, and even medicinal, owing to the stimulus of salt used to cure them. But woodcocks and snipes must not be eaten early in the spring, being then unwholesome. The breast of the pheasant is always safe. Of shell-fish, crabs and oysters are the only species allowed. Lobsters are inadmissible. But there is no objection to trout, sea-bass, rock bass, black-fish, sheepshead, perch, flounders and whiting. Let everyone afflicted with sick-headache be assured of the fact that water is the best diluent and throw aside wine, spirit and malt liquors.'

But despite the almost puritanical attitude of many of our forefathers to alcohol and a deeper understanding today of the physiological and psychological effects of this substance on our body, along with one of the highest tax levies on alcoholic drinks in the world, alcoholism in Britain is still a serious problem in this modern society.

One can recall with a smile the sad experiences of Thomas Burton, 'purveyor of cats' meat to the Lord Mayor and Sheriffs, who has a wooden leg; finds a wooden leg expensive, used to wear second-hand wooden legs, and drink a glass of hot gin and water regularly every night—sometimes two. Found the second-hand wooden leg split and rot very quickly, firmly persuaded that their constitution was undermined by the gin. Buys new wooden legs and drinks nothing but water and weak tea. The new legs last twice as long as the others used to do and he attributes this solely to his temperate habits (triumphant cheers).' (Report of the Committee of the Brick Lane Branch of the United Grand Junction Ebenezer Temperance Association—*Pickwick Papers.*)

However, alcohol does have a direct action on the tissues of the body, affecting both the tissue structure and its functions. Generally when one speaks of alcohol one means ethyl alcohol (C_2H_5OH) but down-and-out alcoholics resort to methyl alcohol, known as methylated spirits and imbibe this in a variety of 'punches', 'red biddy' and 'jungle juice'. When methyl alcohol is taken in large quantities, abdominal pain, vomiting and loss of vision (due to damage to the optic nerve) occur, with eventual death from a toxic coma.

The effects of ethyl alcohol are well known. Initially excitatory, there is at first a stimulant effect on mood and intellect, with free speech and loss of psychological inhibitions that eventually promote amourousness, sentimentality, aggressiveness or depression (depending on the person's basic character and the environmental factor). Judgement becomes impaired and the memory faulty. As the blood level continues to rise the cerebellum, which co-ordinates the movements from the cerebral cortex, becomes affected and purposeful movements become more and more erratic, disturbance of balance, giddiness and ataxic gait follow, leading to eventual unconsciousness. Death may ensue if the alcohol level continues to rise or vomiting and subsequent inhalation occurs. Since alcohol is one of the few substances that is directly absorbed from the stomach (most other substances are absorbed through the small intestine) a recently eaten meal, especially if it contains fatty foods, will slow down absorption. The level taken by the Road Traffic Act to be admissible is 80 mg. per 100 ml. which as almost every drinker knows is equivalent to two and a half pints of beer) above which level, faulty judgement and loss of driving technique will tend to occur. Alcohol also promotes the formation of urine, acting as a diuretic. Thus water taken with alcohol (intermittently as lemonade, etc., or directly mixed, e.g. whisky and soda) is rapidly excreted and will also aid the elimination of the alcohol which has already entered the blood stream.

The after-effects of alcohol are also well known! These are due mainly to dehydration and gastro-intestinal irritation. Dehydration of the cells in the body is due to the loss of water which is required for the renal excretion of alcohol. This gives a dry, furred tongue, sensation of thirst and pounding headache. These after-effects would be much less prominent if it was generally known that by drinking water during or after an alcoholic night out, the cells are rehydrated. A pint of water at the end of a party should be sufficient and repeated if the sensation of thirst begins to appear. The water could be flavoured with fruit juice, etc., to promote palatability. This imbibed water passes directly into the cells of the body and should not appear as increased urinary output to disturb the night's rest. Gastric upset is due to a direct irritant action of ethyl alcohol on the delicate lining of the stomach, producing an excessive outpouring of acid. Alkalis (e.g. aluminium hydroxide solution) or simple milk drinks will neutralize this acid and prevent irritation. Milk, because of its fat content, also slows down absorption of alcohol. The acute diarrhoea which follows alcoholic excess is partly due to a direct irritant action and partly to an allergic response by the bowel—for many beers and wines contain fermented products and particles of yeast that can sensitize the delicate lining of the intestines.

In 1968 there were eighty thousand convictions for offences involving drunkenness, and it is now estimated that there are three hundred and fifty thousand alcoholics in Great Britain. However not every person who drinks excessively is dependent upon alcohol and is thus a true alcoholic. The most widely accepted definition is that offered by the World Health Organization (W.H.O.) 1951.

'Alcoholics are those excessive drinkers whose dependence on alcohol has attained such a degree that they show a noticeable mental disturbance or an interference with their smooth social and economic functioning or who show the prodromal signs of such development.'

'Every morning when I woke up I was sick. I was ill. My hands were so shaky that I'd have to lift the first drink to my lips very, very carefully, to make sure it wasn't spilled. I'd be in such a nervous state, that when I got to the pub I'd sit at the bar and have the first drink while staring in the mirror to make sure no one would come up behind me suddenly. Sometimes in the morning the sweat would be pouring off me, and when I woke up I'd have the heaves, so that even cleaning my teeth would make me retch,' was one case recently reported.

Some drinkers do so to relieve pain, boredom or loneliness. Others do so in bouts, the dipsomaniacs, some continue to drink despite being aware of the accumulative destructive effect alcohol has on them (for example the cirrhotic of *Hobson's Choice*) while others have the classical inability to abstain.

'I would drink in the mornings, a craving, unremitting, that would continue the whole day through, until I had consumed two to three bottles of spirits. Sometimes I would vomit, and sit in the toilet and drink and vomit continually.'

It is often difficult to determine when a person stops drinking like a normal individual. The presence of blackout and amnesia (loss of memory during a drinking episode) the withdrawal symptoms of nausea, 'heaves', tremors, sweating and anxiety that are allayed by the first drink, the continued craving that leads to an increased consumption of rough wines, cheap ports, spirits and ciders—are all pointers to alcohol dependence.

The treatment of an alcoholic by medical means is of paramount importance. Many alcoholics will drink themselves to death, their brains will show increasing degenerative changes and cell loss leading to alcoholic dementia and delirium tremens, when pink elephants, scorpions and headless monsters become a reality. Classically the liver is also severely affected, along with the nervous system, and alcoholic hepatic cirrhosis is well known—the hob-nail liver of the old physicians, so-called because of its irregular, noduled surface. Finally chronic malnutrition and vitamin and protein deficiencies ensue, leading to further mental and physical damage.

The treatment resides in specialized psychiatric centres and hostels, with aversion therapy from drugs as a useful adjunct. Supportive therapy may be needed for many years, especially amongst the truly skid-row alcoholics who frequent the bomb-sites and derelict houses for these often relapse.

Alcohol does produce a withdrawal syndrome if given to healthy volunteers, and from that point of view can be looked upon as a drug of addiction. However, whether it produces profound, irreversible changes like the more serious 'hard' drugs is open to doubt. There is no doubt that many persons who have a regular free access to alcohol—publicans, brewery workers etc. can consume vast amounts of spirit and ales without ever becoming truly addicted. Deep within the alcoholic there lies a psychological personality disturbance that must be corrected before this problem can be overcome. With the availability of alcohol the problems of the reformed alcoholic are immense.

'*Αριστον μὲν ὕδωρ*,' said the Greeks, 'water is best.'

SMOKING—THE DEADLY HABIT

GIVING UP smoking was the easiest thing in the world to Mark Twain who said he had done it hundreds of times. Last year over 32,000 British people gave up smoking. They died from lung cancer. Surgery and radiotherapy is powerless to stem the tide. Only ten per cent of the sufferers will survive, providing they are diagnosed early enough. Many more persons wheeze and pant about the land with their bronchitis and angina. Throw away that shredded weed! The alternative is to light the paper before retiring—to the grave. It is as serious as that! While you read the next few pages someone will have died from lung cancer. It happens every fifteen minutes; six times during a football match; almost one hundred times a day. And this is not the only damage smoking inflicts on the body. More people suffer from, and lose work through chronic bronchitis than any other disease—a disease of smoking, air pollution, industrialization and overcrowding. But who would live almost continually in a thick bluish-grey smog? Only a smoker. The smoker's cough, the early morning sputum are the heralds telling of inflamed airways, proliferating mucus glands and the ultimate destruction of delicate lung tissues. Certain cells in the lungs retain the carbon particles, which is why old miners' lungs were as black as the coal they hewed. The smoker, however, runs additional risks, amongst these being blindness from optic nerve damage, ulcers in the duodenum and stomach, increased risk of coronary thrombosis, giving birth to smaller babies and gangrene of the fingers and toes from vascular damage. These are the simple bonuses of lung cancer and chronic bronchitis. (Incidentally, it causes the elastic tissue in the skin to degenerate faster than normal, thus producing ageing. This fact should cause concern to every woman who smokes.)

What is the evidence linking smoking with lung cancer? Could medicine be wrong? Does giving up smoking have any long term benefits? Does the frequenting of smoky places such as cinemas and pubs carry any dangers?

Hand me my lyre!—as Nero said when he retired to the hills to avoid the risk of bronchitis from the smoke and flames of Rome as it burned.

To start at the beginning. Many years ago (in the early eighteenth century) Percival Potts, the celebrated London surgeon, described chimney sweeps' cancer. This occurred principally on the scrotum. The unfortunate youths, doomed to crawl up chimneys, were thickly ingrained with soot which formed little rounded balls in the natural folds of the body. The irritation produced caused skin cancer. 'Many chimney-sweeps die in youth, few live to the age of fifty,' wrote Thrackrah in 1831.

At the same time other observers were noting an increased incidence of scrotal cancer in the men who worked the spinning Jennys. The prevalence of this—known as Mule Spinners' Disease—was due to the heavy lubricating oils dripping down from the machine on to the spinners' trousers and soaking the crutch.

During the early part of this century two Japanese workers, Yamagiwa and Ichikawa, showed that the application of tar to the skin could produce a skin cancer in rabbits. Later, extracts of oils and soot did the same. The carcinogenic effect was traced to a variety of substances with a certain molecular structure, notably an anthracene ring. One of these, benzpyrene, exists in the smoke of cigarettes (1 mg, per 100).

These substances have also been found in the atmosphere

and statistical investigations in many countries have shown that the death rate from lung cancer is higher in urban than in rural areas, in the ratio of at least two to one, and in some districts may reach the figure of six to one. It is difficult, however, to interpret the effects of atmospheric pollution in such a clear-cut manner, for in densely populated areas cigarette smoking tends to be heavier than in rural districts and also even non-smoking members of the public are exposed to a greater concentration of cigarette fumes in places of entertainment and on transport than those living in the country.

In Jersey, where there is almost a negligible amount of air pollution, the death rate from cancer is as high, if not higher, than most other areas of England and Wales. Similar series on the continent have shown a closer correlation between mortality and smoking than mortality and air pollution.

Deaths from lung cancer have a higher incidence in Great Britain than in any other country, which is not purely related to cigarette consumption, since South Africans and Australians, for example, smoke as much but have a lower mortality rate. When British people emigrate to these countries their death rate from lung cancer still remains higher than the European stock born there. Thus there exists some factor related to the early environment of the British that makes him/her more susceptible to this disease. Of course, Britain is a thickly populated and highly industrialized country and acute and chronic chest infections are commoner here than elsewhere. For years chronic bronchitis was referred to as the 'English disease' and all the evidence available strongly associates atmospheric pollution with chronic bronchitis. The British citizen may also have genetic factors which, coupled with environmental factors (smoking and atmospheric pollution) makes him/her more susceptible to lung conditions, especially cancer.

Occupational factors play an important part in the initiation of lung cancer. The earliest example was recognized in the last century, among workers in the Schneeberg and

Jachymov mines in Czechoslovakia, where there was a high level of radioactivity from the ores obtained, chiefly nickel, cobalt, arsenic and uranium. These mines are still being used behind the Iron Curtain but no information is obtainable from the Communist governments.

Asbestos workers have a higher than normal level of lung cancer and strict regulations and precautions are in force in those industries using this substance. But other people are at risk, chiefly pipe laggers and insulators in the building trade. The inhalation of the fine, short, spiked particles of asbestos leads to destruction of lung tissue and shortness of breath, called asbestosis. (Other similar diseases are silicosis in quarry workers, pneumoconiosis in miners.) However, the inhalation of asbestos dust over a long period leads to a rate of lung cancer roughly fifteen times greater than the general population incidence and the types of cancer produced may be one specific variety peculiar to asbestos inhalation.

In the chromate industry the death rate from cancer of the lung may be twenty-five times the normal, and workers in the distillation of coal in the gas industry and workers with hot tar, continually breathing in fumes heavily laden with cancer-producing polycyclic hydrocarbons, have an increased incidence. Workers in certain metal refining processes, notably nickel refining, which has arsenic as an impurity (and arsenic is a weak cancer substance), have a slightly higher death rate from lung cancer. Through constant supervision and research many of these industrial processes have been modified or eliminated and workers are often moved around to prevent the prolonged exposure necessary to produce cancer. But, despite all the human endeavour and accomplishment in the industrial sphere, lung cancer continues to rise *pari passu* with smoking habits. In the early years of this century the disease was comparatively rare, partly because only a small percentage of the population smoked and partly from poor diagnostic facilities available to the medical profession. Then the population tended to die much younger, the average life span being around forty-five years; the chief killers were infections in infancy and tuberculosis in middle life. The registered deaths from lung cancer in 1900 stood at 273, and 390 in 1910. This rose to 500 by 1920. However, at this period of our history diagnostic aids began to be used more commonly, although this does not completely explain the threefold increase of deaths (1,489) in 1930, a decade later. By 1940 the figure was 5,267; by 1950, 12,000; by 1962, 24,000 and by 1969, 32,000. Since 1940, when females began to smoke more heavily, their death rate from lung cancer has started to accelerate in exactly the same proportions as that of men. Female deaths in the three years 1959-62 rose by twenty-one per cent.

Cancer of the lung reaches its peak in the fifty to sixty age group (average age fifty-seven) but is not unknown in the twenties, more common in the thirties and increasingly so in the forties. Males are affected more than females in the ratio of six to one but certain statistics suggest it is more lethal when found in the female.

Non-smokers are affected by lung cancer but the risks among heavy smokers over the age of forty-five is fifty times as great as for non-smokers. The types of lung cancer found in the non-smoker have not varied a great deal over the last twenty years, whereas two cell types now predominate in smokers, especially one called squamous cell. The death rates from all forms of cancer, other than lung, have fallen by seven per cent from 1950 to 1965, but during this period deaths from lung cancer have increased by seventy-three per cent. Only among doctors has the number of cigarette smokers decreased. In fact less than half the doctors in this country now smoke (forty-two per cent) and correspondingly the death rate (up to 1966) had fallen by seven per cent, regarding lung cancer, which follows the national average for other cancers mentioned above.

Among the doctors on whom this survey was carried out and who were thought to be reliable regarding honest confessions of their smoking habits, the smokers had a twenty per cent greater mortality than non-smokers and if twenty-five or more cigarettes were consumed in a day then the death rate rose by sixty-three per cent. However, among those who smoked only pipes or cigars the excess mortality was one per cent. The mortality mentioned above, age for age, is an overall death rate from smoking, including lung cancer, but does not solely relate to lung cancer, as it includes increased mortality from mouth, throat, larynx and oesophageal cancer, some bladder and prostatic cancers, heart disease, chronic bronchitis and peptic ulcers and cirrhosis of the liver.

Of importance is the fact that by giving up smoking the chances of dying from lung cancer decrease dramatically. The mortality rate is almost halved by five years discontinuance and after fifteen years is only twice the very low rate of non-smokers. However, the risk of a man aged thirty-five *dying* from lung cancer, if he smokes twenty-five or more cigarettes a day, is one in twenty-three in the next ten years and his chances of dying from lung cancer before retiring is one in fourteen, and before he is eighty one in nine.

Smoking is a deadly habit! Death from cancer of the lungs is most unpleasant: death from heart disease and lung troubles most prolonged. There is no remedy to combat this war—a war that loses daily almost as many as were killed in the tragedy of Aberfan—other than prevention. Give up smoking, a relatively simple answer, and doctors are leading the way. If only ten per cent of the present smokers gave up this habit nearly four thousand lives would be saved a year from death by lung cancer alone. When one considers perhaps another forty-seven thousand people that die per year from diseases associated with smoking, the figure would be staggering. Evidence has shown that those born in the British Isles carry through their lives greater risks from smoking than natives of other countries. Since medicine cannot identify those people who will be at risk (apart from those with a smoker's cough), preventive measures must be aimed at the whole population. It seems strange that the public outcry against a few cases of typhoid fever, curable in most cases with antibiotics, and against the food additive cyclamates should be so vehement while the ravages of smoking go almost unheard of and unnoticed. The indulgence in 'hard and soft' drugs and the effects of alcohol on driving make front-page news, while in comparison the seven thousand deaths a year from motor accidents is only a trickle compared to the torrent from smoking. Thirty million working days are lost a year from bronchitis, thirty odd thousand deaths occur every year from lung cancer and the coffers of the Inland Revenue continue to bulge with the revenue from the cigarette industry. If the time between contracting lung cancer and first smoking was short, say a few months, legislation to ban cigarettes permanently would not be long delayed: yet ten or twenty years is relatively short to one who has lived them. Smoking is a deadly habit, noxious, self-inflicted, rightly called the greatest hazard of our time.

THE BLACK DEATH

The Great Plague of 1348-9

FROM A disease which is a scourge of modern times to one which killed nearly half the people in England in the fourteenth century:

I have been told that in the last plague at London, none of the tobacconists' shops had the plague. It is certain that smoking was looked upon as a most excellent preservative, insomuch that even children were obliged to smoke. And I remember that I heard formerly Tom Rogers, who was a yeoman-beadle, say, that when he was that year, when the plague raged, a schoolboy at Eton, all the boys were obliged to smoke in the school every morning, and that he was never whipped so much in his life as he was one morning for not smoking.

Thomas Hearne, Diary, 1721.

English morale, vigour and enterprise had never been higher than during the early part of Edward III's reign. The four million inhabitants enjoyed a new prosperity; vast quantities of fine wool, leather goods, metal ware, coal and lead were exported to the continent and magnificent buildings rose, rich in architectural design. But it was not until the summer of 1346 that England began its ascent to greater glory. On a warm showery evening in France the English army met the most powerful ruler in Christendom supported by counts from Germany, Spain and Luxembourg. Forty thousand soldiers (including seven thousand Genoese bowmen and some of the finest knights in Europe under the banner of Philip VI) swarmed out of the forest of Crecy and pressed home their attack with trumpets sounding and a great cry echoing down the valley. Thirteen thousand Englishmen patiently waited, the setting sun shining on their backs. While the enemy still were outside the range of any contemporary weapon the English archers opened fire and almost fifteen thousand dead were counted in those fields on the misty morrow. The total English loss was forty dead; the longbow now ranked as the supreme weapon of war.

This astonishing victory stirred the English minds and tales of courage and chivalry were passed from village to village. Meanwhile, a far more deadly foe stalked mankind and began its sinister march across the continent. From China came distant reports of earthquakes and floods of terrible magnitude. Arising out of the death and putrefaction came a new and alarming disease: leaving three million dead in China and depopulating vast stretches of India, Tartary and Mesopotamia. Then it spread into the Black Sea area, and via traders into Europe. A contemporary author, Gabriel de Mussi, described how a horde of Tartars besieging the city of Caffa, caught 'the death', as it was called, and realizing that sooner or later all must fall victims to it, turned their vengeance on the besieged and catapulted all their dead over the walls and into the city.

Both the Black Death and the Great Plague of 1665 have been ascribed to Pasteurella pestis, transmitted by the rat-flea from rats to man. Gui de Chauliac, the Pope's physician, stated that 'the epidemic was of two kinds, the first marked by constant fever and blood-spitting from which the patient died in three days, the second with swellings and carbuncles under the arms and groin from which many recovered'. Emperor John Cantacuzene reports: 'Some people died suddenly, others during the course of a day, and some but after a few hours. Those who lingered for two or three days commenced with a violent fever. Soon the poison mounted to the brain, and the sufferer lost the use of his speech, became insensible to what was taking place, and appeared sunk in a deep sleep. The organs of respiration became quickly inflamed, there were sharp pains in the chest, blood was vomited and the breath became foetid. The throat became black and the tongue congested with blood. Those who drank copiously experienced no more relief than those who drank little. The few who recovered had no second attack, or at least not of a serious nature.'

During the first Great Plague of Rome, in the reign of Romulus, we read in Plutarch that it seemed to 'rain blood', a portent which in barbaric ages has several times been recorded. The red fungus which presented this appearance were called blood-spots or signacula. They were observed in the plague of the sixth century and during those of 789 and 959. George Agricola in the sixteenth century pronounced the spots to be caused by a lichen but they gave great alarm to the superstitious folk of medieval times because the sign of the cross could be recognized in these blood spots and the disease seemed like a punishment from God.

The epidemic reached Europe in the early days of 1348, three stricken vessels having put into a port in Genoa in January. From here it spread rapidly. The terror increased when it was found that even the effects and clothes of the dead were capable of communicating the disease. Four unsuspecting soldiers carried back with them a bed-covering they had found in Genoa and slept under it all night for warmth. The next morning all were found to be dead—still huddled beneath. None was spared and twenty-four doctors died in the first outbreak in Venice. Such was the terror that 'the sick man languished alone in his house and none came near him. The most dear to him withdrew, the doctor did not come to him, and even the priest stayed his distance. Men

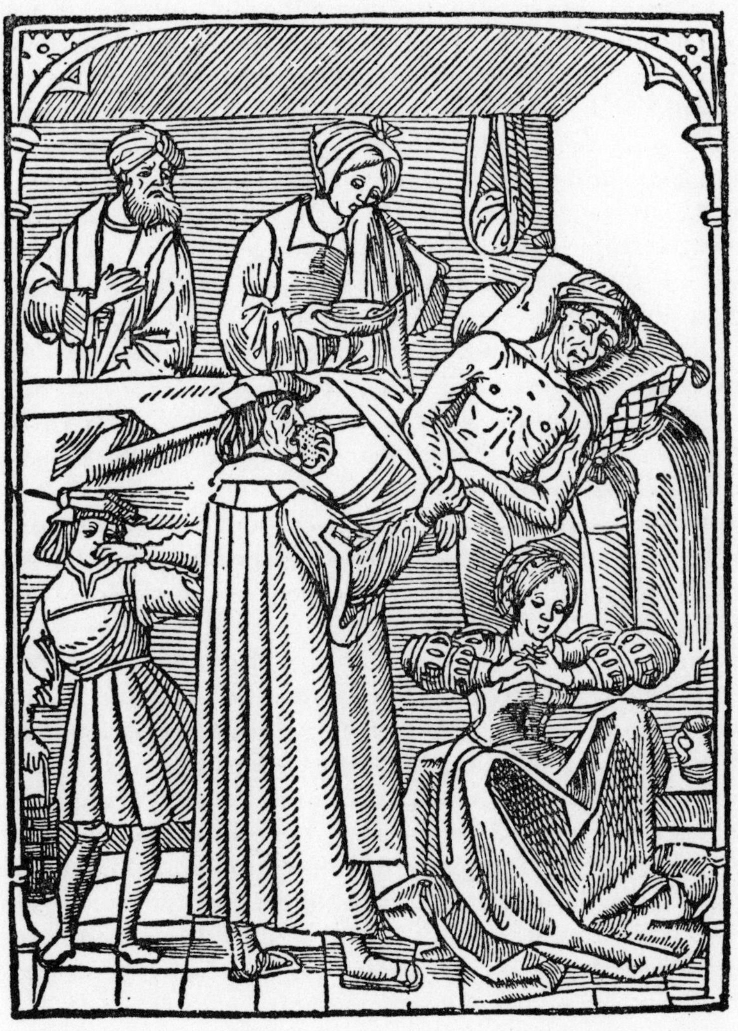

The Plague Doctor. *15th Century*

and women, racked with the consuming fever, pleaded in vain for a draught of water. The father or the wife would not touch the corpse of the child or husband to prepare it for the grave.' 'I could tell dismal stories of living infants being found suckling the breasts of their mothers after they had been dead of plague: and mothers taking up her child that had died and lay'd it in her bosom, by which she was infected and dy'd with the child in her arms also' (Defoe, 1666). 'No prayer was said, no solemn office sung, no bell was tolled. By day and night the corpses were borne to the common plague pit without rite or ceremony. The doors of the houses now desolate remained closed and no one cared, nor indeed, dared to enter.' Some men led a temperate life, avoiding every excess, others feasted and drank. People became selfish and uncharitable, studiously avoiding all infection. Medicines of no value were sold at exorbitant prices and the victims died drinking it—as did the doctors. Desperation gripped everyone, whole families were cast together in the same pit, and God was said to sleep.

Through March and into July the plague marched across Italy, leaving hundreds of thousands dead, and into France. Fifty-seven thousand died in one month in Marseilles alone, ninety thousand in Florence. Covino, a doctor in Paris, wrote: 'A touch, even a breath, was sufficient to transmit the malady.' 'In any house when a person died,' remarked another author, 'all others were attacked and quickly followed him to the grave, even the dogs, cats, cocks and hens also died.' The 'Black Death' continued its spread across Europe until roads became blocked with the dead, and fields and towns were filled with the stench of decomposing bodies.

The summer of 1348 was said to have been the wettest ever in England, and the Leicester chronicler, Henry Knighton, attributed this to the wanton behaviour of ladies at tournaments. Despite every precaution, the plague crossed the Channel and, in August, came the dark tidings that the infecion had broken out in a Dorset coastal town of Melcombe

Regis (now Weymouth). Here most of the inhabitants were destroyed, and sweeping over the southern districts, it destroyed numerous people in Dorset, Devon and Somerset. 'It passed,' writes the Registrar of Canterbury Court, 'most rapidly from place to place, swiftly killing ere mid-day many who were well in the morning. On the same day forty, sixty and very often more corpses were committed to the same grave.' Before the close of 1348 the pestilence had spread itself far and wide in the western counties of England. In Bristol 'living were scarce to bury the dead', such were the numbers that survived; and the people of Gloucestershire would have nothing to do with Bristol men, but the unsuspected rats ran from town to town. Thus the disease reached Gloucester, Oxford and London, leaving only one-tenth of the population behind, and in the narrow streets the grass grew several inches, high, fertile and undisturbed. New burial grounds were consecrated, fields left uncultivated, food prices rose, and the poor faced starvation.

Owing to the speed at which the plague slew, the worse was over in the south before it reached the Midlands and North in the spring of 1349. Taxes, fines and tithes remained unpaid and at one court held in Houghton (near Durham), it is recorded 'that there is no one to who will pay the fine for any land, which is in their lords hands, through fear of the plague'. In Northumberland in 1353, six hundred pounds was still owing to the King in taxes for twenty-five parishes. So many merchants and rich people died in Newcastle that it also could not pay its dues The plague did not reach Alnwick until the spring of 1350, and the Scots, 'hearing of the pestilence, laughed at their enemies and thinking that a terrible judgement of God had overwhelmed the English, assembled in the forest of Selkirk with the intention of invading. But alas, the "terrible mortality" came upon them and within a short time died five thousand'.

The number of persons who died in the 'Black Death' can never be fully calculated, but estimates from deaths amongst the clergy and other sources put the number in England between one-third and one-half the population, roughly two million deaths. Some villages, like Tilsgarsley in Oxfordshire, and Middle Carleton in Leicestershire, were never reborn. The price of food, the shortage of labour and the deaths of many aristocratic and land-owning families had repercussions on the English social system for many decades to come. But although the plague abated in the early 1350's, for three hundred years it would periodically flare up, and the red cross on the door, the cart piled with corpses, the pit for the stricken, and the cry of 'Bring out your dead!' would reappear once more to disturb the life of a rapidly developing land.

GONE TO THE DEVIL

A Study of Ancient Witchcraft

THE DESTRUCTION of one quarter of the population as the Black Death swept Europe in the fourteenth century led to a culminating wave of terror. The Victory of Satan seemed near. Whole devout congregations disappeared and the few clergy that remained were sunk in apathy and despair. For the first time great numbers began to see in the Devil a new cult, a new creed. Witchcraft became a philosophy with a literature of its own. Similar rites, similar ceremonies sprang up all over the world; common bonds and customs independent of race or language made the supernatural a grim and vital reality to all mankind.

Then came the Papal Bull of Innocent VII and the notorious Inquisition, determined to eradicate to the last trace all witchcraft in the western world. In 1489 Sprenger and Kramer, Inquisitors of considerable energies, published their great textbook *Malleus Maleficarium* (The Witches' Hammer) and the most ferocious wave of torture and human suffering was instituted with the approval of Pope, Church and layman alike.

The origin of the witch is lost in pagan antiquity. She emerges out of the dimness of the primitive world as the wise woman, adapted by the Bronze Age men as the Great Mother Goddess, the principle of fertility, the source of all life. Since she was skilled in home and field the broom and pitchfork became her sacred symbols of the faith. To her spells and incantations the sick and infertile turned. But if the Bronze Age man had one strength, it was his one fear. Without his metals he was weak, a victim of wild beasts and neighbouring tribes and for these metals he needed fire, flames that had to be jealously guarded, nurtured, protected, with almost divine affection. As men were required to hunt they could not be spared for this task, so in time the women were selected for this duty. These women had to be separate from the child-bearing group, however, and virginity became a prerequisite factor. Later the same train of thought was reflected in Greek and Roman mythology as the vestal virgins.

With the advent of Christianity the old gods were driven into the darkness and their priestesses were transformed from wise women into witches, the Vestals' hearth becoming the sympathetic origin of the cauldron. However, the advent of Christian healing embodied some of the principles and drugs used in witchcraft. Self-hypnosis and auto-suggestion, the juices of the poppy, deadly nightshade, henbane, hemp, all became an integral part of early medicine. Meanwhile the Church continued to pronounce on the sickness of the body as the visitation of the Devil. More and more the mournful ideals of mortification and victory over death by the humiliation of the flesh were preached from the pulpits, and supported by excerpts from the Bible (Exodus, xxii, 18). More and more the people turned to the charlatans and witches as the Christian medical methods failed. Superstitious medicine held sway and the idea that strange parts of animals held magic properties became rife. Cocks' combs, cygnets, ants' eggs, frogs' spawn, jaws of pikes, perspiration, saliva, body hair, internals of hens, woodlice, were the pharmacopoeia of the day. As the feudal oppression of the early Middle Ages deepened, the fatal philosophy of the witch, with her secret arts and potions, became welcomed to alleviate the terrors and beliefs of the peasantry.

What was a witch? Gifford (1857) defined her as 'one that worketh for the Devil, hunting or healing, for telling things to come, which the Devil has devised to snare men's souls to damnation'; Sabbat ... was a nocturnal assembly of witches, necromancy ... the revelation of hidden treasures and other practices by calling up the devil in the likeness of one who has died, Incubus ... a lewd demon who sought sexual intercourse with a woman, exorcism ... the driving of a devil out of a man. The most important activities included the pact when witches undertook to blaspheme and desecrate the Host, to defile corpses, to commit sexual offences, to pervert and corrupt, as in the Devil's war against the Church. Ointments allowed witches to change their form or fly. Disasters, such as floods, tempests, the death of a farm animal, destruction of crops, etc., were their domain. While in the realm of sex and perversion, nightmares were the visit of a sexual demon or 'mare' whose icy touch left the victim cold, terrified and exhausted.

But not all were ugly, ageing hags. In fact the very terms 'bewitched', 'charming', 'enchanting', emphasize the fact that many were seemingly beautiful girls, leading normal lives, secretly performing as witches until suspicion fell on them. For suspicion meant confession and confession meant death by fire.

The most common and tragic side of the trials was the conviction by personal evidence or confession. To the courts a witch was a witch until she was proved guilty and then she was destroyed for the benefit of the human race. Prisoners were allowed neither witness nor defending counsel, for these then would automatically be regarded as supporting heresy and be in turn condemned to Hell's eternal flames. Church witnesses were allowed to be anonymous. The Inquisitor would plead with the victim, trying to get him to confess. If this measure failed, he was then submitted to torture of the most primitive and barbaric kind. This was carried out in carefully controlled stages. The prisoner was first hoisted up a ladder, his limbs being strapped to the rungs so that his frame was stretched to capacity. Thumb-presses were then applied to convert the tips to a pultaceous mass. Weights were attached to his feet and he was allowed to jerk suddenly so that part of his spine dislocated with a snap. Vices were then applied to the limbs, nails driven into the bone marrow and, before the final burning, the victim was given a foretaste of hellfire by having a hot iron or pincers thrust on to the throat or tongue. Luckily for English witches they were usually hanged, although the occasional one was boiled. An ancient clinical trial was immersion in water—if the victim floated she was guilty. In this the accused was stripped of all but a single garment and bound hand and foot, crosswise. In this helpless condition she was thrown into the water, sometimes with a rope around her waist as a precaution against drowning. If she sank, she was innocent but, as so often happened, she floated, her guilt was proved because the pure water had rejected one who in turn had rejected the water of baptism. The following case was reported at Hertford Assizes. Thomas Colley was condemned for the murder of Ruth Osborne (his wife) near Tring. The populace, having feared a witch in the neighbourhood, 'wrapped the wife and her husband in two different sheets, first tying their great toes and thumbs together, the most active of the mob dragged the woman into the water by a cord which they had put round her body, and she not sinking, the prisoner Colley went into the pond and turned her over several times with a stick; after a considerable time she was hauled to shore, and the old man was dragged into the pond in the same manner; and this they repeated to each three times. The woman, after she was dragg'd in the third time, being pushed about by the prisoner, slipped out of the sheet and her body was exposed naked; notwithstanding which the prisoner continued to push on the breast with his stick, which she with her left hand endeavoured to catch hold of, but was prevented by his snatching it away. After using her in this manner till she was motionless, they dragg'd her to shore and laid her on the ground, where she expired.'

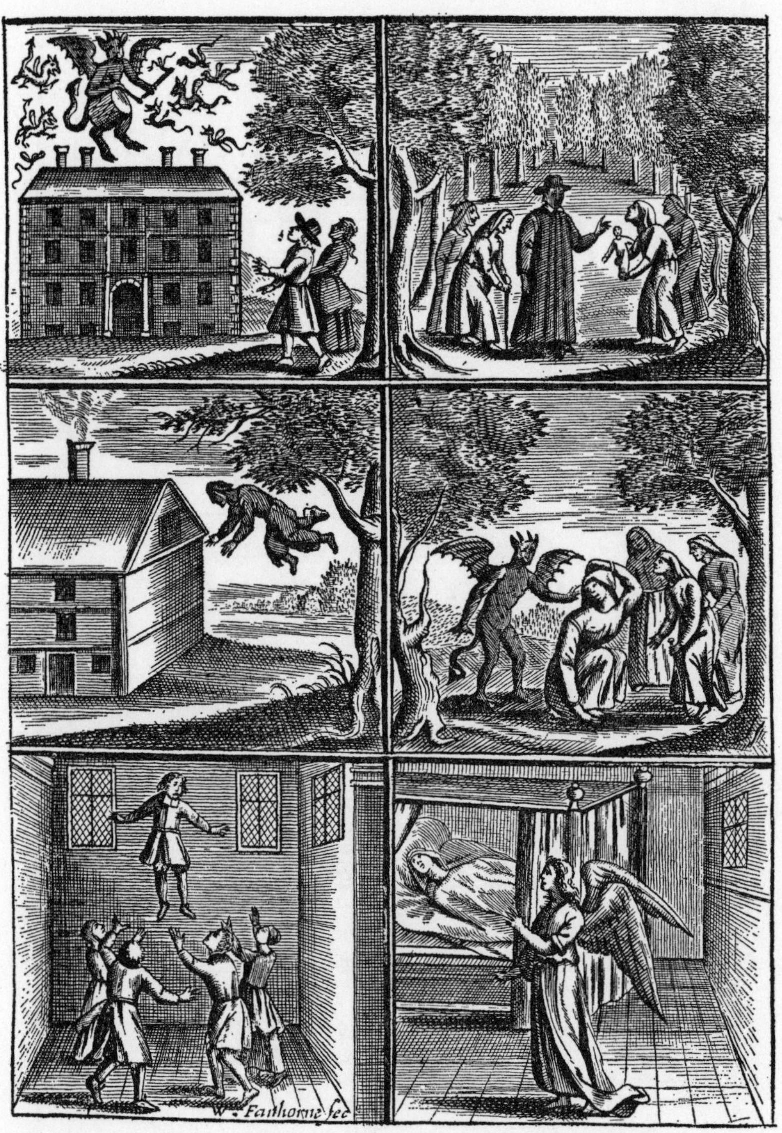

Witchcraft *W. Faithorne*

Saducismus Triumphatus:

OR,

Full and Plain EVIDENCE

Concerning

WITCHES

AND

APPARITIONS.

In Two PARTS.

The First treating of their

POSSIBILITY;

The Second of their

Real Existence.

By *Joseph Glanvil*, late Chaplain in Ordinary to His Majesty, and Fellow of the Royal Society.

The Third Edition.

The Advantages whereof above the former, the Reader may understand out of Dr *H. More*'s Account prefixed thereunto.

With two Authentick, but wonderful Stories of certain *Swedish Witches*; done into *English* by *A. HORNECK*, D.D.

London, Printed for *S. L.* and are to be sold by *Anth. Baskervile*, at the *Bible*, the Corner of *Essex-street*, without *Temple-Bar*, M DC LXXXIX.

Witch trials were lucrative for judges, witnesses and torturers, since the victims' families had to pay all the costs, and a good supply of witches was always to be found, especially in Scotland! Rapidly introduced from the Continent was the Witch-finder who spread fear throughout the towns and villages he visited, being always amenable to a bribe of any kind. In the north of England they received twenty shillings a head and some finders specialized in investigating young women whose husbands were eager to get rid of them.

The German Rhineland and the Swiss states exceed all others in savagery and the list of condemned is proof of the terror that captured the medieval imagination. At Treves seven thousand are said to have been burned, six hundred by a single bishop in Bamberg, nine hundred in Wartzburg, while one judge boasted of killing eight hundred in sixteen years and another nine hundred; four hundred died in Toulouse in one day. Scotland was close behind with four thousand, four hundred burnings but this was still insignificant when compared with a hundred thousand in Germany. England shows a relatively moderate score, less than a thousand being condemned to death. The last execution for proven witchcraft was in Germany in 1775, the last in Ireland in Tipperary in 1894.

Many of the accused suffered from mental illness; some were simply the victims of a social prejudice or malevolence. The most important illnesses were, of course, schizophrenia, epilepsy, depression and delirium due to malnutrition, G.P.I. and inborn errors of metabolism. The persecution of the witch was not so much the expression of the sadistic nature of a few warped individuals but the outcome of religious ideals, socially orienated to protect mankind from a long and lingering hellfire; for only true witches were 'sent to the Devil'.

Take 'twenty garden snails which be in shells, beaten, in morter, until you perceive them to come to a salue, will bothe heale a bile and drawe it. A drop or two of a iuyce of a black snail, dropped on a corne will take it away speedile. A wine of earthworms, with a little scraped ivory and English saffron, will do a man who has the iaundice "maruellous much good". Earthworms are also an infallible test in the diagnosis of kings evil. Take a ground worm and lay it upon the place grieved, then take a green dock leaf or two, and lay upon the worme, and then binde he same about the neck of the party diseased, at night when he goes to bed, and in the morning when he rises, take off againe, and if it be the kings euil the worme will turn into powder or duste. For the cure of whooping cough take a mouse and flea it, and drie it in an oven, and beat it to powder, and let the partie drink it in ale, and it will help him.' From Dickens' Household Words.

'The chips off a gallows on which several persons had been hanged, when worn in a bag around the neck, would cure the ague, a stone with a hole in it, suspended at the head of the bed, would stop nightmare, hence it was called a hagstone, as it prevented witches from sitting upon the sleeper's stomach. The same amulet tied to the key of a stable door, deterred witches from riding horses over the countryside. Headache was cured by the moss growing on a human skull, dried and pulverized, and taken as cephalic snuff. A dead man's hand could dispel tumours of glands, by stroking the part nine times, but the hand of a man who had been cut down was most efficacious.'

FAITH

The brute necessity of believing something so long as life lasts does not justify any belief in particular
(*Santayana*)

FAITH CAN move mountains, is on the road to revelation merges darkness into light and, as Cardinal Newman said, 'It is faith that makes martyrs.' What is faith and what are the physiological and psychological adjustments necessary?

The acquisition of faith can be an isolated experience like that of St. Paul on the road to Damascus, St. Cuthbert in the northern hills or a mass phenomenon like the meetings of John Wesley and the Nuremberg rallies of Adolf Hitler but these recipients have one thing in common. They suddenly and uncritically accept a doctrine alien to their previous beliefs and stick to this doctrine unshakably, although this may often be based on an illogical conclusion. Let us examine this sudden acquisition of faith.

Firstly, as John Wesley inferred, it may occur when the mind is mentally prepared by being in a state of extreme fear, anxiety or unremitting mental conflict. This can be amplified by the hypnotic effect of mass movement, participation and rhythmical singing. By dwelling on and magnifying the Lord's wrath, the subservience of man, his many inadequacies, idolatry, wretchedness and the inherent sin of all, Wesley was able to produce the required background of mental and emotional confusion and thus provide an atmosphere conducive to the indoctrination of his faith. The huge propaganda machine of Goebbels converted the German peoples in precisely the same manner in the 1930's. Then, the thunder of drums and marching feet, the packed, cheering arenas, the hysterical emotions released were as effective in this political conversion to a misplaced faith in a human being who was regarded as a god, as evangelical missions were, and still are, effective in the indoctrination of faith in the Christian God. But in turn these techniques are as old as man himself, for in the primitive state man turns to the voodoo gods, totems and wild spirits and the worship of these involves dancing and singing, accompanied by the steady and methodical rhythm of drums, which finally builds up to a frenzied crescendo of movement and noise to become so overwhelming to the participants that a trance is created during which the spirits of good or evil enter or leave the victim's body at the will of the medicine man or priest. Men and women under such suggestive conditions can be induced to perversion and crime but often the trance is used as an emotional outlet to free the physical and mental being of unwanted illness and ideals, leaving the victim exhausted but content. The early settlers in Mexico and South America used a variety of drugs to obtain the same hallucinatory effect, among them mescaline and LSD. During the trances evoked the persons involved would offer themselves to their gods, chiefly Aztec, giving their hearts and perhaps other organs as sacrifices to the altar.

The means of conversion by fear and excitement are basically the same when used to create new faiths in political meetings, or religious revival groups. Often the faith is incomprehensible to anybody not experiencing the whole effect and the part it plays in the convert's mind is out of all proportion to its real value. Nothing is more tedious than the convert, fired with acquired zeal, preaching his ideals at every opportunity.

So far I have discussed only mass conversion occurring under the influence of rhythmic repetition of stimuli and in an emotionally charged environment. But in other creeds, for example the doctrine of Zen Buddhism, contemplation is necessary for long periods in quiet solitude, with the mind acting as a mirror to reflect all extraneous thoughts and sensations, devoid of all passion and emotion of any description. The Indian fakir on his high pole is active mentally, if not physically. Many other faiths adopt similar attitudes and were common in the medieval period of our history in the monasteries and abbeys that abounded. Several hermitages still exist today, handed down by our pious forefathers, where people once isolated themselves from the sins of the world for mystical contemplation.

Scientists studying the mechanism of faith often quote the classical work of Pavlov, the Russian physiologist. He found that when his dogs were subjected to two complementary stimuli at the same time, for example the ringing of a bell and the application of food, the dogs soon learned to salivate when the bell was rung alone. However, once, when a flood had destroyed the kennels and almost drowned the animals, he observed not only a complete cessation of previously acquired reflexes, but the substitution of new ones (in the illustration above the dogs might, for example, show aggressive behaviour). Thus he believed the nervous system could alter in relation to its appreciation of its environment and might, after an initial frightening experience, go into a state of emotional blunting, to be followed by a period when previous positive responses became negative and vice versa, i.e. a complete alteration in likes and dislikes. Thus the subject's whole outlook on life becomes coloured from another spectrum and feelings of possession by other beings or faiths become manifest and the new impressions, despite being at total variance with the subject's background and previous beliefs, become deeply imprinted in the subconscious, dictating future thoughts and actions.

But are the new faiths permanent? On many occasions the answer must be yes. However, time can destroy suddenly induced ideas, although the period of removal is much slower than the period of acquisition. Drugs can be employed to alter a patient's outlook and electric shock treatment, brain operations and indeed brain injuries can also have an eliminating effect.

In some people, however, faith remains untarnished and a spiritual guide for good or evil. As Tolstoy said, 'Faith is that by which we live.' In this day and age, is it?'

PSYCHEDELIC DRUGS

THE PROBLEM of drug addiction has mushroomed during the last decade and although the seriousness of the situation in Britain does not approach that of other western countries, notably the United States, it does give rise to considerable anxiety among those of the medical and political professions. Unfortunately there is always a minority of individuals in society who, because of their mental instability, social inadequacies or disrupted family life, are always prone to drug taking. The main concern is not for this hard core but for the many young persons at universities, colleges and in other groups who experiment with drugs, often at the instigation of seasoned addicts, and who do not fully realize the potential danger of these compounds. While we have another vociferous minority, some of whom are in responsible positions in academic life, who continually praise the soft drugs as a means of emotional release, the difficulty of persuading the adolescent to avoid drugs will become increasingly greater. Alcohol is now accepted in society, with all its inherent dangers of addiction, crime, sexual release, etc., but there is no reason why other substances capable of promoting the same antisocial behaviour, such as hashish, should be released into the community, also bearing in mind that a great number of hard addicts begin on these so-called soft drugs.

Drug addiction is associated with both mental and physical deterioration; the average span of life of a heroin addict is in the region of five years.

So what factors drive a young person to drugs. According to Blaine 'A number of young drug users feel, usually with very little evidence, that they are sexually abnormal and that some drug will enable them to engage in more satisfactory sexual relations. The recent trend towards beginning sexual intercourse at an earlier age has put added pressure on teenagers for performance before many of them are physically or emotionally ready for it. Their failures lead some of them to reach false conclusions about impotence or frigidity. Such fears have caused a few to search for a drug which can impart instant sexual maturity.

A few hope that a drug will actually change them, but many more are convinced that taking drugs will make friends for them. People smoking pot or taking LSD are under the impression that they communicate more meaningfully and as a result they believe that happy and fulfilling alliances will follow. Nonparticipants at such gatherings report little is said. The individuals involved spend much of their time giving descriptions of the effect of the drug as it works on them, but in general the smokers are just as isolated as at other times.

Most youthful drug takers are experimenters, those who enjoy meeting challenges and taking risks. Many are motivated by rebellion or hostility which they express by breaking rules. Some, the oblivion seekers, find the drugged state of mind a pleasant respite from the stresses of the world. In attempting to explain their decision these people point to the injustices in our society. Most of those who purport to be 'dropping out' are burdened by a feeling of incompetence and guilt. It is not that they do not believe in success, but that they do not feel they can achieve that success. Some, attempting to bring about a basic change in personality, feel compelled to combine drugs and to escalate dosage as disappointment and frustration mount.

The principal potent psychedelic drugs are LSD, Mescaline, Psilocin, Bufotenine, Dimethyltryptamine. Marihuana is a milder member of the hallucinogens. The term psychedelic means 'mind manifesting' and is broadly applied to a variety of substances, materials and events in this enlightened day and age. Although the hallucinogens are relatively new in the clinical and experimental fields of medicine the plants from which these drugs are derived were familiar to ancient civilizations. The Vikings chewed a poisonous type of mushroom before battle to obtain the desired warlike effect it produced on the mind. The Aztecs used hallucinogenic mushrooms and peyote in their sacrificial ceremonies. Even today some Indians continue to use peyote buttons—the dried, cut-off tops of the peyote cactus, in their religious ceremonies. Of course man has always been willing to experiment with plants and certain very valuable substances (for example, digitalis, was discovered from the foxglove and aspirin from the willow). Many other substances, if used properly, have a valuable role to play in medicine, notable examples being atropine from the deadly nightshade, and morphine, opium, papaverine, etc., from the oriental poppy. The pleasant effects of opium have been known for thousands of years and can be produced by eating or smoking it, drinking extracts or injecting the purified, active principles. The word opium is Greek for juice and originated in Turkey, which still produces a great deal of opium, but its introduction into India, China and the Far East has done a great deal of harm.

Cannabis indica, or hemp, hashish, marihuana, bhang, dagga (they are all the same) has already been referred to as a so-called soft hallucinogen. The drug is prepared from a resin which is found on the flowers and stem and on the leaves of the hemp plant, which is an annual herb closely related to our hop and is grown as a crop for the sake of its inner bark which is used for making twine, thread, rope and canvas. Hemp seeds are also used as bird food. The man who has chewed, swallowed, or smoked hemp appears at first dull, then fatuous and excited, before he finally goes to sleep. Moreau de Tours in 1845 was one of the first to study the effects of hashish on normal and highly gifted subjects. He concluded that the fundamental aspects of mental illness could be reproduced by the use of this compound. During intoxication with hemp the concept of space and time are grossly distorted so that minutes seem like hours, colours become more vivid, pain is lessened and the mind races uncontrollably from one subject to another with many bizarre ideas. Indian hemp is said to lead to crime and the very word assassin was first applied to the Muslim sect of the time of Saladin because they carried out murders under the influence of hashish. Alcohol was forbidden by Mohammed!

Certain scholars have regarded the hallucinogens as an important aid in man's effort to achieve a greater understanding of himself and the world he lives in. Introspective studies on the effects of peyote (mescaline) were recorded by Weir Mitchell and Havelock Ellis, (also by Aldous Huxley in *Doors of Perception* and by D. H. Lawrence in *The Woman who Rode Away*).

The most significant effects of the hallucinogens (or psychedelic drugs) have been outlined above in regard to hashish. However, the accompanying emotional reaction may vary from elation, excitement, depression, anxiety or a variety of mood changes, during the period of intoxication. The type of emotional reaction appears to be influenced by the dosage of the drug, the basic personality of the individual, the surroundings and company in which the drug is given, Following the use of LSD, the hallucinations and depersonalization may re-occur for weeks or even months after it has been given up.

The exact mechanism whereby these drugs affect the brain, and their site of action, is not fully worked out. It is thought they block the metabolism of key chemical substances like serotonin and histamine in the brain and release others like noradrenaline and adrenaline. The fact that persons under the influence of the hallucinogens behave in some cases like schizophrenics lends support to the idea that this disease is due to defective metabolism in the brain, resulting in the build-up of substances in composition or nature similar to the hallucinogenic drugs.

Much publicity attends the popular cult of drug taking, especially LSD, to 'improve the mind', 'expand the consciousness', 'get with it' and for 'kicks' in the hippy cult of 'drop out' and 'social rejection' to avoid the responsibilities of modern living. Admissions to certain hospitals have shown that of the acute psychoses due to LSD, the average age was twenty-two and the main symptoms were: an overwhelming fear, uncontrolled, violent urges with strong auditory and visual hallucinations. There was a high incidence of attempted suicide in these patients. The majority recovered in two days but in an unfortunate few the symptoms persisted for a prolonged period and required long term hospital admission.

This cult is rotten so let's get rid of 'the beast/the hawk/the chief/the ghost/crackers' (some slang terms for LSD) and also the 'bad seed/button/tops/full moon/big chief' (slang for peyote and mescaline). Let's stick to Mars Bars and milk—and get fat!

SLEEP

O Sleep! it is a gentle thing,
Beloved from pole to pole!
To Mary Queen the praise be given!
She sent the gentle sleep from Heaven
that slid into my soul.

Coleridge

SLEEP IS essential for normal animal and human survival but the quantity and quality of sleep differs between species and among individuals of the same species. Animals deprived of sleep die after a few days. Ancient Hindu observers recognized two levels of sleep, dreaming (paradoxical) and dreamless (light) sleep and until recently the normal mechanism and body alterations occurring with sleep had not been investigated. Lucretius surmised that the fidgeting of animals during sleep were linked with dreams. Klaue, a German, recorded the wave disturbances of the brain on an electroencephalograph some thirty years ago. He found that sleep progressed in a characteristic sequence; a period of light sleep, during which the waves produced by the brain were slow, followed by a period of deep sleep, during which all activity was speeded up. More recent observers have found that during this period of rapid wave production the eyes moved rapidly under closed lids. Further investigations revealed that dreaming is always associated with the rapid-eye-movement (R.E.M.).

Among animals the pattern of sleep varies. The European

swift (Apus) actually sleeps on the wing; bats and flying foxes can only sleep when their heads hang down and they are suspended by their feet and certain whales close only one eye while sleeping and switch off the corresponding half of their brain. This had been closely observed in the dolphin when the period of sleep for each eye was up to three hours. Among fishes and reptiles, who possess no eyelids, sleep is only for relatively short periods and a sudden light can cause alarm when introduced into an aquarium or reptile house at night. In birds the state of sleep lasts no longer than fifteen seconds at a time and comprises less than one per cent of their lives, as compared with twenty to thirty per cent in higher animals. However, birds do dream, for paradoxical sleep occurs in their very brief periods of sleep. All mammals studied by Jouvet, from a mouse to a chimpanzee, are found to dream. The hunting animals (cat, dog, wolf, man) enjoy a deeper sleep with more dreaming than do the hunted (rabbits, hares, deer, etc.). The former spend twenty per cent of their sleeping time dreaming, the latter five to ten per cent. For many years it was considered that many of the hunted animals, especially the ruminants like cattle and deer, did not sleep, but recent observations have shown it to be of a short duration (five to ten minutes). Most animals sleep well only in a secure environment—the hippopotamus half submerged in water, the fox in his den, the mouse snug in his mouse-hole. Birds instinctively try to reach the highest point in a tree for sleep, or hide in the thickest bush or secluded nook of a building. Fully grown birds sleep outside the nest during the mating season as a rule, the exceptions being the sparrow and woodpecker. Among the higher animals—the anthropoid apes—a high vantage point in a tree is sought. Gorillas, orang-utans and chimpanzees build new nests every evening. In most of the creatures mentioned, vision is reduced by closing the eyes and by shielding them by some means such as using the paws or tail (fox, husky etc.). In some animals, notably the bat family with their very large ears, the outer part is folded to reduce sound perception.

Thus sleep has appeared among animals late in the evolutionary process. But the pattern is not rigidly fixed at birth; for example, a newborn kitten spends half of its time in the waking state and half in paradoxical or dreaming sleep, going directly from one to the other without light sleep intervening. By the end of the first month the capacity for light sleep has become acquired and in the adult state it occupies fifty per cent of the animal's time, with fifteen per cent dreaming or paradoxical sleep and thirty-five per cent awake. Thus a cat spends almost two thirds of its life sleeping, curled up in a ball with its neck bent. This bending (or flexion) of the neck denotes tone (Jouvet) and light sleep. After twenty minutes or so the neck and back relax, the curvature is lost as the muscle tone vanishes, the eyes move rapidly in a variety of directions and the muscles of the body may show slight tremors, the paws may move slightly, the whiskers, tail and ears twitch and the breathing becomes irregular. After six or seven minutes the light sleep with slow brain waves re-occurs and lasts for a further twenty minutes.

The control of sleep in all mammals, including man, is probably diffusely scattered through the brain, with interplay of impulses from the arousal centre found in the midbrain and known as the reticular formation. Many substances produced in the body, especially under stress, like noradrenaline and serotonin, affect the arousal centre and produce long periods of wakefulness. Sleep disturbances due to anxiety or worry may have a similar cause.

There is no set limit for the amount of sleep people need. Some individuals claim never to sleep, while others manage on two to three hours per night. The average is about seven and a half to eight hours. All persons, however, require a certain amount of dreaming sleep. If deprived, (by an experiment so that they receive a small electric shock when rapid eye movements appear, which wakes them up) they will rapidly revert to dreaming, when allowed to sleep normally again and

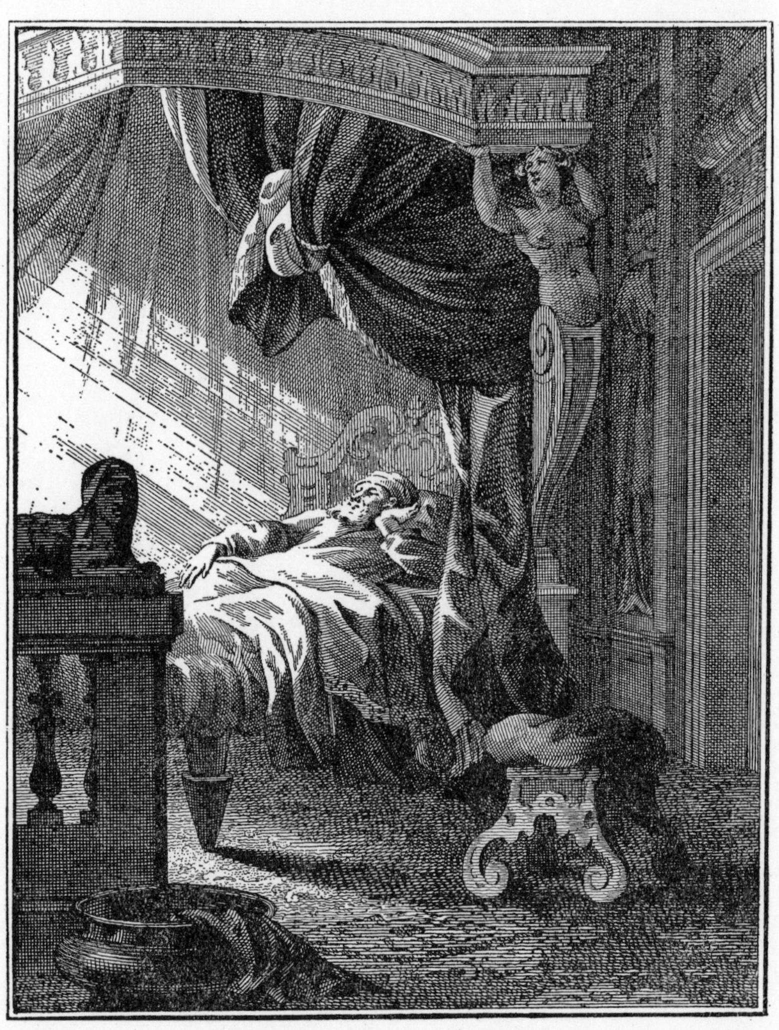

Man Asleep. *R. Vinkales*

will dream longer and more vividly. Thus nature seems to determine that a certain percentage of dream sleep is a necessity. Many drugs prescribed by doctors to promote sleep only produce the light variety of sleep and the person wakes unrefreshed and still tired. The best treatment for sleeplessness remains a quiet, darkened room, a period of exercise beforehand and a warm beverage taken prior to retiring. But some people just do not require all the sleep they try to obtain and their anxiety to sleep further interferes with rest. A series of late nights in a relaxed environment (e.g. holidays) often breaks this period of sleepless nights.

Sleeping is a complex, physiological phenomenon, which has inspired poets for generations but only the medical profession recently and presumably there is a great deal still to discover about that state in which we spend such a large part of our lives.

The sun descending in the west,
The evening star does shine;
The birds are silent in their nest,
And I must seek for mine.

Blake.

THE SEVERED HEAD

M. Hendrich, the headsman of Paris, and indeed lately of France, is dead, having discharged the duties of his office for no less than fifty-four years. During this period a hundred and thirty-nine criminals passed through his hands. He was once asked by a visitor whether he thought the separated head continued to live after it had rolled into the basket. He pondered a few minutes, as if to collect his memory, and then related instances which went to support an affirmative answer. Among them he said that on one occasion a woman's head made a faint effort to spit at him; and he spoke of violent contortions occurring in the muscles of Orsini's face. Similar contractions were observed to occur in Queen Mary's face after decapitation. But none of these movements can be regarded in any other light than as of the nature of reflex actions. The stimulus, no doubt, is the sudden loss of blood which here, as elsewhere, induces convulsions, and we repudiate the idea that consciousness is preserved even for a moment in the decapitated head.

Lancet, nineteenth century.

But, according to Pinel, the body dies quietly and painlessly from haemorrhage in the course of a few minutes, but the brain, being shielded from atmospheric pressure, retains its blood, and consequently life, for a long period. The sources of common sensation are indeed cut away, but the nerves of hearing, sight and smell remain, and the whole apparatus of consciousness and intellect is present. Dr. Pinel paints the horrors of a situation which, according to him, may last as long as three hours.

It is true enough that the brain does retain a large quantity of blood after decapitation, but it is equally certain that the blood rapidly becomes venous from lack of oxygen, and experiments have amply proved that, in complete asphyxia, consciousness is entirely abolished in one minute and a half, and is, of course, being progressively lowered during the whole of that time. But, considering the tremendous physical shock which is inflicted by decapitation, it is nearly certain that all nervous function must be paralysed too completely to allow of any phenomenon of consciousness taking place during the short period necessary for the perfect de-oxydization of the blood in the brain, after which mental action can never be resumed. At the most, the suffering after decapitation by guillotine can only be an affair of moments.

Lancet, nineteenth century correspond.

Much has been written, and many conflicting opinions expressed, as to whether the head after severance, retains any sensibility, and the question has been revived in Paris appropos of Lemaire's execution. M. Bonnafont gives the following account of an experiment on the dissevered heads of two Arabs, which will probably put the question to rest. He says, 'I was in Algiers in 1833, where I met with a military surgeon who asked me about this question. I then heard that on the following day two Arabs were to be beheaded, and obtained leave to make conclusive experiments on the subject. For this purpose I had placed on the execution ground a small, low table, on which was placed a large shallow vase, nearly filled with powdered plaster. I then went to the place of execution with a small ear trumpet and a very sharp lancet. It had been agreed that the charus should place the head, immediately after it was cut off, upon plaster of Paris to stop the haemorrhage. M. Fallois was to speak to the heads by name, placing the ear trumpet to the ear, while I examined the eyes and other features. This was done, but notwithstanding all the shouts into the ear, I could not perceive the slightest sign of life. The eyes remained glassy and motionless, the face discoloured.'

B.M.J.

There is no doubt that after execution, either by guillotine or hanging, the body dies immediately. The sudden shock received by the nervous elements in the vital centres of the medulla (a region of the brain just above the neck) causes instantaneous loss of consciousness and death. Any activity occurring afterwards is simply of a reflex nature due to cells of the brain discharging their energy before dying.

The medulla and other 'lower centres' of brain activity occupy a large percentage of the brain substance; the activities of locomotion and the associated sensations, perceptions and thought processes are found in the cerebral cortex. Damage to this area, by a motor accident for example, can produce permanent loss of movement, sensation and consciousness, while the other parts of the brain function normally to keep the individual 'alive'. On the continent the concept of brain death is recognized. (See Transplantation, page 131.)

SUICIDE

'Will you dine with me today?' said a Frenchman to a friend. 'With the greatest pleasure: yet, now I think of it, I am particularly engaged to shoot myself: one cannot get off such an engagement.' This is not the suicide à la mode *with us. We ape at no such extra refinement or civilization. We can be romantic without blowing out our brains. English lovers, when the course of true love is interrupted, do not retire to some secluded spot and rush into the next world by a brace of pistols tied up with cherry-coloured ribbons. When we shoot ourselves, it is done with true English gravity—it is no joke with us.*

That the disposition to commit suicide may occasionally be hereditary is shown by Dr. Burrows cases. 'I have observed several members of one family, where there is a propensity to commit suicide, declare itself through three generations: in the first, the grandfather hung himself; he left four sons: one hung himself, one cut his throat and the other drowned himself in a very extraordinary manner, the fourth died a natural death, which, from his eccentricity and unequal mind, was scarcely to be expected. Two of these sons had large families; one child of the third son died insane; two others drowned themselves, another is now insane, and has made the most determined attempt on his life. Several of the progeny of this family, being the fourth generation, bore strong marks of the same fatal propensity.' The English are not, par excellence, a suicide people. When the inhabitants of a country are prudent and industrious, the crime of self destruction will be rare.'

Dr. F. Winslow on suicide, nineteenth century.

Eleven persons in every hundred thousand commit suicide, males only slightly more than females, with a marked increase over recent years in the younger age group, especially between twenty and twenty-five. However, the preponderance is in the elderly.

Sleeping tablets and tranquillizers are the most popular vehicles in this modern age, while deaths by violent means are usually only found in the most severely depressed and often have a marked exhibitional quality associated with them. Occasionally spectacular cases are reported. These consist of blowing up 'planes or buildings, with the loss of many innocent lives as well. Other sensational techniques involve the murder of famous people; for example some psychiatrists have suggested that Oswald, President Kennedy's assassin, comes into this category.

A word of comfort. Suicide ideas are very common, even among people free from psychiatric symptoms. Most people imagine themselves as Ophelias floating on a bed of flowers into tranquillity, during some period of their lives, but this daydream bears *no* relation to intent.

Even among people who have attempted suicide the likelihood of future attempts varies greatly. Some people make weekend habits of taking minor overdoses just to occupy a niche in a hectic Casualty Department on a Saturday night. Others are genuinely in need of assistance, if only temporarily, and their attempt at suicide is a cry for help. There are high risk groups, however. Suicide, despite the recent increase in younger persons, is very much a condition of later life. Then it is related to social isolation (I feel like repeating this word), retirement, lack of employment, loss of friends and relations, failing health and finally loss of status in society and the home. Depression does not always accompany suicide in old age, but a history of a broken home in childhood is commoner even in the aged who commit suicide.

Other high risk groups are as follows: unskilled workers are more prone than skilled workers but the professional and managerial classes have the highest incidence. In these people social pressures accumulate, and fear of social decline, failure, dampened aspirations ultimately precipitate a crisis. Higher suicide rates are found in university students than in their contemporaries in commerce and industry. As far as students are concerned, it is higher in those who follow a non-vocational course than in those who seek a career in medicine, for example, while separation from home is another salient factor. It is to be noted that psychiatric disturbances, mostly neuroses, are the commonest illnesses interfering with academic life.

The prevention of suicide needs a rational approach to protect the individual against the suicide impulse. This implies medical and social intervention if there is any risk whatsoever. Doctors should be able to recognize the early alterations in mental attitudes, especially in the groups referred to, priests can aid in the home by sorting out family and social problems that have gone beyond the capability of those concerned, and such services as the Good Samaritans play an invaluable role in the immediate treatment of the suicide subject. However, because only one third of the people who commit suicide are mentally ill in the true sense of the word, the removal of stress and the formation of stable human relationships is a dominant factor in prophylaxis.

To conclude, let me once more mention the people who deserve special attention from doctors, clergy, relations and friends. People who talk about suicide never do it. Rubbish! They, and those persons having previously attempted suicide, need careful observation and guidance. The rate is highest in densely populated areas, widowhood, divorced states, alcohol and drug addiction, broken childhood homes, physical illness, mental illness, economic stress, childlessness and social isolation.

Rural living, religious fervour, lower socio-economic class, a large number of children and the married state (!) are all associated with a decreased incidence of suicide.

Today, more than ever before, economic stresses and social isolation are to be found among an ever-ageing population, and the risk of suicide increases. Do you know any old person who lives alone? So many of the present generation do not seem to care.

THE NAKED APE

THE NAKED APE? ... Full marks for ape, but man has actually more hairs per square inch than any chimpanzee and during development in the womb is among the hairiest of animals. So, is the nakedness of man a vestigial feature, as certain authors would suggest, or is it another product of man's advanced evolution? The answer is simple. Man has the largest brain in the animal kingdom and the brain is roughly divided into two compartments, motor and sensory. The numerous fine hairs that are to be seen in profusion over most of the body are richly endowed with fine nerve endings, consisting of nearly two million sensory antennae. A vast number of impulses are transmitted to the brain every second by these fine hairs. Try ruffling them with a pen and see. This complex sensory apparatus constantly links us with our external environment.

Some areas of the body are truly naked. These include the palms of the hands, the soles of the feet, a small area around the upper and lower lips and certain parts of the genitalia. These regions are the most sensitive parts in the body and the amount of brain given over to them is disproportionately large. Try a simple test. Take two fine points on a drawing compass, diverge the points and try and detect at what distance between them only one single prick can be experienced. On the fingers this will only be a millimetre or so but on the central region of the back, a relatively insensitive area, the difference may amount to a centimetre or more.

It is interesting to compare the skin on the two surfaces of the arm. The front or flexor surface is relatively naked but the back or extensor surface is more hairy. The skin is much thinner on the flexor surface and in consequence the fine nerve endings reach closer to the surface and are correspondingly more sensitive. Burns and superficial wounds that leave the raw nerve endings exposed are very painful. Thus evolution (or Nature, call it what you will) has gradually shed the coarse cumbersome hairs, to replace them with a fine layer infinitely more suitable for the environment in which man now exists. In this respect, women seem to lead the way!

The sensations from skin contact are transmitted from infancy, through sexual life into old age. A baby's experience through its skin, of being fondled and caressed, appears vital for its subsequent development. Such fondling precedes visual and perhaps auditory stimuli (although certain reports indicate that a baby listens to the mother's heartbeat while in the womb and is soothed and comforted by it in its first few months of growth. Watch how most mothers instinctively hold the infant with its head against the left [or heart-beating] side of the chest. It isn't simply due to right-handedness).

The joys of mutually sought skin contact shared with a loved one are among the advantages gained in terms of evolutionary nakedness. In shedding coarse, dense hair, scales and thickened skin man finds freedom to exist in a more truly sensitive environment and demonstrates once more the hidden subtleties of evolution.

Footnote: Finger nails are found on the dorsal surface of the finger in direct apposition to the pulp which is the most sensitive area in the body. Pressure on the pulp deforms it against the nails, which thus amplifies the sensory stimulus. So nails are more than effete hoofs or ornamental vestiges.

THE MAGIC BULLET

or How the First Germ War Was Won

'HAVING SEVERAL times endeavoured to discover the cause of the pungency of pepper on the tongue; I did put about one third of an ounce of whole pepper in water, placing it in my study. The pepper having lain about three weeks in water I looked upon it the 24th April, 1676, and discerned in it, to my great wonder, an incredible number of little animals, of divers kinds . . . were incredibly small and so small in my eye, that I judge if a hundred of them lay one by another, they would not equal the length of a grain of coarse sand, and according to this estimate, ten hundred thousand of them could not equal the dimensions of a grain of such sand.'—Antony Leeuwenhoek (1632-1723), lived in Delft and his hobby was lens grinding. He made this startling observation in 1676, but its exact importance was unrealized for more than two centuries.

'Living things are produced by the union of some passive principle, "matter and an active principle", "form", this form being the soul of all living things. Matter or substance by itself is devoid of life but is vivified by the energy of the soul. The soul is present in varying amounts in the elements—earth, water, air and fire—of which living things are made, and their relative amounts control the nature of the life endowed by the soul. Thus the earth endows plants, water, aquatic animals, and air terrestrial forms. The form of living things originates from their like depends on animal heat but the form of those arising spontaneously from matter depends on the sun's heat. Slime and decaying matter might possess some soul but do not of themselves produce living organisms, the fructifying influence of rain, air and heat being required for the *spontaneous generation of life.*' So wrote Aristotle (384-322 B.C.): his teachings profoundly influenced the fathers of the Christian Church and led to the acceptance of the theory of spontaneous generation by the Church. To disbelieve was heresy.

'God maketh wine from water and earth by the grape, but our Lord Jesus maketh wine from water. In like manner He can cause the living creatures to be born from seed or matter containing the invisible seed.' Thus St. Augustine (354-430) also lent weight to the spontaneous generation theory, while medieval scholars corroborate these ideas with fantastic observations and experiments of their own.

'Place a dirty shirt in a vessel containing wheat and after twenty-one days storage in a dark place, to allow fermentation to be completed, the vapours of the seeds and the germinating principle in human sweat contained in the dirty shirt will generate live mice.'—Van Helmont, alchemist and physician (1652).

The Greeks firmly believed that decaying meat could, together with air and warmth, give rise to small white worms.

'Between the meat and flies I placed a screen of muslin, so that, although the air did circulate freely, and that the meat decomposed, yet no worms appeared.'—The Italian poet/physician Redi (1668). He concluded that the decaying matter merely offered a nest for the flies' eggs, and that the white worms were nothing more than flies' larvae.

About this time we return once more to Leeuwenhoek and his lens grinding. By the clever use of phase contact microscopy he observed blood corpuscles, spermatozoa and microorganisms for the first time. He found that it was only necessary to place readily decomposable matter in a warm place for it to become teeming with small creatures. He held the revolutionary idea that they arose from animals already present in the material, in the container, or in the air in contact with the material. His follower, Joblot, found that by boiling such infusions for fifteen minutes they would no longer give rise to additional germs if stored in a closed container. When the cover was removed, however, new microorganisms appeared. 'In the air near the surface of the earth there fly or float innumerable quantities of very minute animals of diverse species which settle on the plants that are agreeable to them and there come to rest, take some nourishment and bring forth their little ones.'—Joblot.

Meanwhile the French biologist, Buffon, and the Welsh priest, Needham, maintained that life 'can originate by spontaneous means in flasks of mutton gravy or other infusions, boiled and stoppered while hot'. 'I took a quantity of mutton gravy hot from the fire and shut it up in a phial closed with a cork so well masticated that my precautions amounted to as much as if I had sealed my phial hermetically. I neglected no precautions. The phials closed or not closed, the water boiled or not boiled, the infusions permitted to teem with animals.'—Needham.

But another Italian, Lazzara Spallanzani, in 1765, entered the arena of spontaneous generation and an acrimonious debate flourished between him and Needham. He criticized the vessels Needham used, the length and degree of heat employed and the effectiveness of the sealed corks. In return Needham contended that Spallanzani heated his infusions too vigorously, thus destroying the special creative force.

Spallanzani was undeterred. His careful investigations showed that fertilization even in mammals could not occur without direct contact of sperm with ovum. For fertilization to be possible therefore it was necessary to accept the existence of an ovum in the female genital tract. He studied fertilization in frogs and toads and noted that when the male sex organs were covered with wax linen, the ova remained unfertile after mating. He collected the liquid in the sac and found that it could induce fertilization. He repeated the work of artificial insemination in a bitch, having collected the sperm from a dog. These experiments became the foundation of the doctrine of generation by male and female cells and nullified some of the dogma that had been accepted for centuries.

In 1836 Theodor Schwann, the founder of the cellular theory, passed air through a heated tube (and later through acids) into a broth that had been boiled, thus supplying oxygen and gases, but the soup did not become infected. Proponents of the idea of a vital force in air claimed that heating or strong acids could destroy this vital force and hence spontaneous generation could not occur. 'When by meditation it was evident to me that spontaneous generation was one of the means employed by nature for the reproduction of living things, I applied myself to discover the methods by which this takes place.' Thus in 1859 Pouchet, in an extensive work of over seven hundred pages, 'showed' that spontaneous generation did occur.

Meanwhile the French Academy of Sciences offered a prize to settle, once and for all, by 'an exact and convincing experiment', the problem of spontaneous generation. This prize was won by a remarkable man, Louis Pasteur, the founder of modern bacteriology.

Pasteur demonstrated that there was a widespread distribution of micro-organisms in the air and concluded that airborne micro-organisms were a chief source of contamination of the broths, juices and various other foodstuffs. One of his experiments consisted of sterilizing broths in flasks with the necks elongated into a tortuous letter S in a horizontal position. In these goosenecked flasks there was a direct contact of the culture fluids with the air but dust and germs settled out in the bent portions of the neck and the fluids remained sterile. Since the air in these flasks was not heated, filtered or subjected to any chemical treatment, there was no chance of the vital force being altered or destroyed—a brilliantly simple experiment from the greatest research worker of all time. Not only did he perceive that certain germs could live without oxygen (anaerobic) as well as with it (aerobic) but he studied the process of fermentation, and was able to show that the undesired odours and tastes in French wine were due to the activity of certain germs. By heating the wine to 55°-60°C. this undesired fermentation was prevented (the process of pasteurization applied to milk today). Research in diseases of silk worms, which were threatening the silk industry, anthrax and rabies all followed, each one brilliantly investigated by Pasteur's analytical and 'farseeing' mind.

The germ theory as the cause of infectious disease was now firmly established. Robert Koch (1882) was a German who became interested in the work of Pasteur; he discovered the cause of tuberculosis and anthrax and made many notable advances in the technique of culture and propagation of bacteria.

Now, during this period of history, surgery was crippled by infection. The mortality from infection was terrific and wounds were expected to fester and become putrid. War surgery, was almost horrific. Paré, the famous French surgeon, when the Duke of Guise was struck with an arrow in the face, 'which buried its head deeply', simply put his foot on the Duke's face and by sheer force pulled the arrow out. Wards were dirty and the stench of corruption almost unbearable. Women were dragged from the streets of Paris, refusing to be taken to the maternity hospital, even though they were in labour, for they knew that almost all caught puerperal fever and died when they were delivered in its filthy surroundings. It was not until the pioneer work of Semmelweis in Austria that washing the hands in a chlorate of lime solution became popular to eradicate transmitted infection. Gangrene, abscesses, septicaemia were rife.

'There is one of my cases at the Infirmary which I am sure will be of interest. It is a compound fracture of the leg with a wound of considerable size and accompanied by great bruising and great effusion of blood into the substance of the limb, causing great swelling. Though hardly expecting success I tried the application of carbolic acid to the wound to prevent decomposition of the blood and so avoid the fearful mischief of suppuration throughout the limb. Well, it is now eight days since the accident, and the patient has been going on exactly as if there was no external wound. His appetite, sleep, etc., is good and the limb daily diminishes in size, while there is no appearance whatever of any matter forming. Thus a most dangerous accident seems to have been entirely deprived of its dangerous element.'—Joseph Lister (1864), the father of antisepsis, introduced his famous spray of carbolic acid during operation and paved the way to sterile surgery.

'No one considers the lion which leaps on its prey to be a parasite nor the snake which injects venom. One creature destroys the life of another to preserve its own. This condition we will call antibiosis (against life).'—Vuillemin in 1889.

For generations, the Mayans had used a fungus known as 'cuxum', growing on green corn, for the treatment of ulcers and intestinal infections. Peasants in the Ukraine had cured septic wounds by the application of moulds and the natives of Brazil had used small green 'puff' balls from the fields to heal wounds.

'It was during a visit through central Europe in 1908 that I came across the fact that almost every farm house followed the practice of keeping a mouldy loaf on one of the beams in the kitchen. When I asked the reason for this I was told that it was an old custom and that when any member of the family received an injury such as a cut or bruise a thin slice from the outside of the loaf was cut off, mixed into a paste with water and applied to the wound with a bandage. I was assured that no infection would then result from such a cut.'—Cliffe (1908).

The moss upon dead men's skulls was also efficacious in the

seventeenth century. Apart from the treatment of malaria by chinchona bark and the tape worm by extracts from ferns, very little, apart from the application of mercury paste and caustics, had been attempted before the twentieth century, although in 1852 Mosse wrote in the *Lancet*: 'Being in practice in the west of England, where troublesome boils rage, I was induced to try common yeast in doses of a tablespoon with some water, three times a day. I have now practised nearly six years and have had the frequent opportunities of witnessing the good effect of yeast.'

'In one of the tubes the Bacteria lost their transitory power, fell to the bottom and left the liquid between them and the superficial layers clear. Six other tubes showed the same muddiness, all of them became quickly covered in mould, under which the bacteria died or passed into a quiescent state and fell to the bottom. The "clay colour" was the slime of dead bacteria, the cause of their quiescence being the blanket of the Penicillium mould.' Tyndall in 1876 preceded the discovery of penicillin by over fifty years.

In 1888 work commenced on injecting rabbits with inoculations of a germ, Pseudomonas pyocyanea, and ten years later workers had isolated a substance that was bactericidal, pyocyanase. It was used with some success, chiefly in diphtheria.

In 1909 Paul Ehrlich's long search came to an end. For years he had believed that certain protein chains would make a bacterium susceptible to a chemical compound without affecting the host. 'The magic bullet', he called the compound. Painstakingly he searched through a variety of chemicals and at the 606th attempt introduced the arsenical substance 'salvarsan' that revolutionized the treatment of syphilis. Later neo-salvarsan (914th) was introduced and proved to be more effective. The 'magic bullets' not only hit the parasite but killed it.

In 1932 two German chemists applied for the patent of a scarlet dye called prontosil, used in the dyeing industry which had an added sulphonamide group to increase its fastness for silk an wool.

Domagk (1935), working with infected mice, found that the animals could be kept alive if treated with this scarlet dye, prontosil. Then came dramatic reports of cures of patients with puerperal fever, by Colebrook and Kenny. The active principle was traced to sulphanilamide and many varieties flooded the market in the late thirties, the best remembered by the term 'M. and B.' (May and Baker). Sulphonamides are in active clinical use even today.

Before this, however, in 1928, a bacteriologist, Dr. Alexander Fleming, observed that when a mould invaded his culture plate of staphylococcus (a common skin germ which produces boils etc.), the growth of the bacteria was prevented over a large area. 'I cultivated the mould and made extracts and tested it. It destroyed the bacteria without any apparent destructive action on the leukocytes. It was non-irritant when applied to the eyes or a wound and it was no more toxic than the nutrient broth when injected into animals. The strength of the broth-culture of this mould was such that it could be diluted to nearly one in a thousand before it lost its powers. It was these observations which stimulated me in my first paper on penicillin to say: "It may be an efficient antiseptic for the application to, or injection into, areas infected with penicillin-sensitive microbes".' Fleming continued to work on penicillin but not being a chemist had little success.

In 1935 Howard Florey, an Australian (later to become Lord Florey), was appointed a professor at Oxford. Working with the German-born Ernst B. Chain, they decided to investigate a variety of substances produced by bacteria.

'The first investigations decided upon at Oxford included a study of penicillin, because it was effective against the staphylococcus, for which no effective remedy was known at the time.' So they reported in 1938. The crude testing methods were improved and a very small quantity of impure penicillin was available for mouse experiments. 'Fortune favours the prepared mind,' Pasteur had written, and fortune favoured Fleming and also Florey and his workers. Had the drug been used on other experimental animals, especially the guinea pig, in this impure form, then death from allergy would have resulted and penicillin would probably have been discarded. On 25th May, 1940, four mice were selected. All four were suffering from a streptococcal infection. The control mice without penicillin died within sixteen and a half hours, the other two continued to live. These two small creatures carried the hopes and welfare of mankind. One survived indefinitely, the other thirteen days. Further mice trials were then arranged and the results were very encouraging. But the amount of penicillin that could be produced in the laboratory was very small. 'The mould would only grow on shallow layers of fluid. Wartime demands made it difficult to secure the needed apparatus. At first old-time circular bedpans were pressed into service, later flat ceramic bottles. Milk churns were used in the extraction apparatus.'—Florey.

'On 27th January, 1941, the first patient to receive an injection of penicillin was given this intravenously, 100 mg. of material being injected. The patient was not suffering from any infection but was a volunteer. She showed no signs or symptoms immediately after the injection but three hours later developed a sharp rise of temperature.'—(Abraham, Chain *et al.*). This temperature was due to the impurities in the penicillin extract.

'On 12th February, 1941, an Oxford policeman, dying of septicaemia, was given penicillin intravenously at intervals. Within twenty-four hours he improved and continued to progress for five days, but then the meagre stock of penicillin was exhausted and the patient relapsed and died. The second was a boy with osteomylitis. His infection cleared for a while. The third patient was a man with a large carbuncle which healed in a striking fashion.' (Florey *et al.*).

To supplement the pitifully small supplies the penicillin

was re-extracted from the urine of the patients who had received the drug.

Finally, because England was still at war, the United States undertook full-scale preparation of the drug in giant tanks, with better penicillin strains and nutrient medicines. By the beginning of 1942 enough material had been collected to start a second series of clinical trials. Of fifteen cases of serious infections treated by penicillin, twelve responded, one fulminating case of meningitis recovered, as did two other lethal infections. The 'magic bullet' had truly arrived and the first germ war was won.

THE CAUSE OF CANCER

PEOPLE OFTEN ask 'What is the cause of cancer?' Let it be stated categorically, 'There is no one cause, but a multitude.' After years of research doctors and scientists are still ignorant about the basic changes that take place in a cell to make it malignant. Once this property has been conferred, however, the cells invade the normal tissues of the body, burning up vital nourishment to produce emaciation of the host, and causing symptoms by pressure and erosion. Not only do cancer cells destroy locally but they float round in the blood, lymph and body fluids and like seeds in the wind, settle in new environments and flourish.

The comparison with seeds is important, for the success of the malignant cells depends not only on themselves but the 'soil' of the host. Every person can develop cancer, but some do so more easily than others. In transplantation the ever-alert white cells are mentioned and it seems in malignant diseases that these cells can and often do destroy the relatively foreign cancer cells. In some cases, for unknown reasons, their ability becomes impaired and the new tissue flourishes to form a tumour.

Cancer tissue grows rapidly and often outstrips its blood supply, so that large areas die and ulcerate, with the seepage of small quantities of blood that herald the clinical onset of the disease. Any bleeding in the human requires investigation and should not be ignored.

However, not all cancers are fatal; in fact, during the last decade almost half the sufferers of cancer were permanently cured, and many persons die of other illnesses before the terminal stages of cancer, since the greatest percentage of patients are elderly. One must not lose sight of the fact that cancer is the second commonest cause of death in young children (accidents being the first).

Much requires to be done, much more money is needed. But progress continues, albeit slowly. New drugs are constantly being introduced, and in some forms of cancer, notably chorionic cancer, a disease of the pregnant uterus, a total cure can be induced by drugs. However, there are many forms of cancer, even a wide variety occurring in one organ, like the lung, and each will probably require a different form of surgical and medical treatment.

As for the causes, these depend on diet, chemical, environmental, viral and racial factors. For example, gastric cancer has a remarkably high prevalence in Iceland. It is also high in Norway and Finland, while the incidence in Japan is five times that of the United States. By contrast, stomach cancer is rare in Java, Indo-China, Nigeria and certain parts of central Africa. But these factors are not purely racial and genetic. Cold to temperate climates affect dietary habits. The Icelandic people have a diet, high in fish and mutton, which is cured by smoking and salting, and some chemicals in these processes may induce cancer. In Finland infestation by a fish tapeworm is common. This creature absorbs valuable vitamins that are essential for the normal function of the cells of the stomach. By contrast the Japanese eat very little fish, mainly subsisting on rice dishes, but stomach cancer is still very common. In the United States there is a lower incidence than in most other countries, the rate being higher in the northern states than in the southern and immigrants are more liable to contract this disease than the native stock. In Britain, North Wales has twice the rate of southern England, and maybe this is related to the presence of trace elements of zinc, cobalt, chromium and the organic content of the soil. It was observed that in one area of Devon, where there were two tanneries using chrome, the mortality rate from cancer of the stomach was greatly increased, whereas in another area of the town without the tanneries, the death rate was not raised above average. The importance of water supply, polluted with materials from the atmosphere, is not fully evaluated, although surface water from shallow rivers, lakes and wells may contain significantly increased amounts of cancer-promoting substances and this could be related to a higher incidence of stomach cancer than normal. But peat soils have a higher level of radioactivity than chalk and limestone and there are many peaty areas in Wales. Lower social classes suffer from cancer more often than the managerial class and in Wales quarry workers and farmers suffer more commonly than any other groups, although the incidence in their wives does not follow this pattern. What are the effects of oral hygiene, tobacco, hot foods, chemicals, infections, vitamin deficiencies, heredity? We do not know! Stomach cancer simply illustrates the complexity of the problem.

However, when one studies the geographical influence on cancer production one finds many fascinating questions and very few answers. In the case of one malignant disease that exists in a peculiar pattern in Africa, several strange features were elucidated by Burkitt in 1958. This disease resembles the leukaemias and is found in children between five and six years old. It is called Burkitt's lymphoma and usually kills within six months. Burkitt observed that the disease did not occur at a certain altitude above sea level i.e. five thousand feet and appeared to be linked to temperature. He also found that the annual rainfall was above twenty inches in high risk areas. With the places involved the altitude limit and the local temperatures closely corresponded to the distribution of certain insects, notably the tsetse fly and some varieties of mosquito. But these creatures do not by themselves induce this lymphoma. A virus seems to be involved, passed by the infected bites of these insects.

Another African distribution of cancer has been studied. This is cancer of the bladder. Egypt has the highest incidence of this and it has been discovered that this is due to the fact that bilharzia, a disease caused by a 'fluke'-like parasite, Schistosoma, is very common. In the Nile valley a considerable number of the population earn their livelihood by farming, using primitive methods and working barefooted in water, where indiscriminate micturition occurs. In the voided urine are millions of small eggs that hatch and, after growing in small snails, leave their intermediate host and enter the unbroken skin. Since religious observance requires ablutions after defaecation and urination, these are carried out at the water's edge, leading to reinfestation of the water by more eggs. Once the parasite enters the veins around the bladder, nodules and warts are formed in the bladder and many cases later become malignant.

In the problem of skin cancer, sunshine is important. In 1894 Unna correlated skin cancer with prolonged exposure to sunlight, being more common in sailors, fishermen, farmers and other outdoor workers. Ultra-violet light seems to be the causative agent. Fair-skinned, blue-eyed and red-headed individuals that freckle and burn without tanning easily seem to be at risk. The tan, due to dark pigmented cells of the skin, has a protective action in screening and shuts out these harmful rays to some extent. Negroes and Bantu races are only rarely affected by skin cancer. However, prolonged exposure is needed over ten or more years, even as late as forty years, before the first changes, a solar dermatitis, are found in the skin. The colour changes to red and yellow/brown patches, with thinning and scaling and occasional deeply pigmented freckles. Eventually warty changes supervene, which may in turn lead to cancer. These changes are commonest on the forehead and cheeks, where solar radiations are most severely felt.

But sunlight is not the only cause of skin cancer. Radiation from the early X-ray machines produced malignant changes in the fingers and hands of the doctors who first used them. Soot and oils initiated skin cancer in the scrotum in the chimney sweeps and leather workers of previous centuries while arsenic in dyes and local remedies produced a dermatitis and eventually cancerous change.

Cancer of the bladder has already been referred to. In 1895 Rehn reported the onset of tumours in persons who worked with aniline dyes and aromatic amines in Germany. When the supplies from Germany were cut off in 1914, manufacturing plants opened in Britain, to be followed by the onset of bladder cancer in their workers. One hundred and one cases were reported in two factories by Goldblatt in 1949. The period of exposure may be short and one workman only worked for a hundred and thirty-one days with these substances before eventually developing bladder cancer. Usually the cancer does not show itself for fifteen to twenty years. However, not all cases of bladder cancer occur in people exposed in industry. Most are spontaneous, their cause unknown. Since any chemical substance excreted in the urine is concentrated in the bladder and retained there for long periods, and the individual is exposed to millions of compounds during his lifetime, the elusive cancer-promoting chemical (or chemicals) may be difficult to track down. Sufficient to say that smoking is associated with treble the risk of bladder cancer.

Of the causes of the cancers outlined above we know a little. Of many other varieties we understand nothing. Thus the research worker turns to experimental animals and wild creatures for help.

Until 1911 it had been found possible to transmit a malignant growth only by means of the living cells of the tumour by transplantations from one animal to another of the same species. In that year Peyton Rous, working in New York, described a cancer of the chicken which could be transmitted by a cell-free filtrate of an extract of the growth or the dried cancer cells. Other workers produced similar experiments in ducks and pheasants. The invisible agent produced tumours more rapidly than chemicals and was present throughout the growth, increasing in amounts with cell multiplication. The causative agent was a virus, varying in size between 30 and 200 μ (5-30,000,000 in one millimetre, or 125-750,000,000 in one inch). Newly-hatched chicks and ducks were even more susceptible to infection by the virus, with increasing age the resistance becoming progressively more marked. Many of the tumours produced were types of leukaemia. Later Gross (1951) succeeded in transmitting leukaemia in a mouse by a centrifuged cell-free solution.

But the next significant observation in animals, after Rouse, was made by Shope, who, in 1935, observed a warty growth existing in wild cotton-tail rabbits in America and found, on investigation, that it was caused by a virus. Later Rous was to show that if tar was applied to a rabbit's ear only a mild, simple growth appeared but if, after a suitable interval, the Shope virus was injected into the rabbit's circulation, then a malignant growth developed at the site of the application of the tar.

The mouse, because of its rapid multiplication and ease of in-breeding, has been extensively used in the study of cancer. One of the most interesting observations came from the experiments of Bittner who found that certain strains of mice continually developed breast cancer. By mating mice of high cancer strain with those of low cancer strain it was shown that the offspring had a high cancer incidence only when the mother was of high cancer incidence and suckled the young. If the mother was of low incidence, with a father of high cancer strain then the baby mice did not develop cancer. Since the offspring in the matings were identical from the genetic point of view, the cancer trait was not passed by genes. If suckling was prevented then cancer did not appear in the baby mice. Further work showed the 'milk factor' to be a small, virus-like particle and only a few drops of milk were necessary to transmit it to the young. Several other viruses have been shown in animal tumours but with the possible exception of Burkitt's lymphoma, none can be proved to be the cause of cancer in man. Certain simple conditions, like the common wart and laryngeal warts, are due to viruses and may regress spontaneously, but they are usually harmless. The antagonists to the virus theory point out that the agent must either be present in the body or in close approximation, e.g. on the skin, and point out that the prolonged period between induction and tumour presentation does not favour a viral origin, which usually rapidly promotes tumour growth. Since most viruses are tissue-specific, then a multitude of different organisms are needed for each variety of cancer. The protagonist of the viral cause of cancer point out the numerous animal tumours that have a viral basis. They say that since cancer is often similar in appearance and progression in man they find it difficult to assume a different basis for human cancer. The problem still remains unsolved, but it appears that viruses may either alone or acting in conjunction with various physical and chemical agencies, produce certain forms of tumour in the human.

I have already mentioned radiation in the causation of cancer. Leukaemia occurred in the survivors of the atomic bomb disasters at Hiroshima and Nagasaki. Cancer of the bones is prevalent in dial painters, who use luminous paint, and in people who have been subjected to prolonged exposure to radiotherapy in the early period of its use in medicine, before proper precautions were taken. There is no doubt that radioactivity, by interfering with the normal division of the nucleus of the cell, is a potent cancer-inducing agent and will continue to increase in importance in this day and age when the radiation hazard to mankind is becoming increasingly severe. The death rate from leukaemia in England and Wales rose almost fourfold during the 1930-60 period and its rate of increase comes third to lung cancer and coronary disease (previously mentioned).

Chronic irritation may lead to cancer. Thus cancer of the

tongue was once common in clay pipe smokers, where the sharp stem of the pipe continually damaged the delicate lining of the lips and mouth. Old scars from burns, tuberculosis of the skin and syphilitic disease, may become the seat of malignant transformation. Cancer of the cervix may be related to the repeated trauma of intercourse and childbirth. Cancer of the stomach can occur in a gastric ulcer (but never a duodenal). The presence of stones in the gall bladder and kidneys for long periods may set up malignant change. Trauma itself does not cause cancer, although a blow on the region may draw attention to a lump, or a fracture may occur through diseased bones. Some cancers can originate in abnormal cells left over from the foetus but are rare and tend to be found in children.

The heredity aspect of cancer worries people whose parents have been cancer victims. The appraisal of the place of heredity in malignant disease has to be viewed against the background of the high prevalence of the disease. Since cancer affects up to one in five people, the evidence of heredity is difficult to analyse and environmental factors come into play. The study of twins has not elucidated the problem. Certain familiar conditions predispose to the formation of tumours. These conditions are genetically determined. Studies of other types of cancer show certain familiar relationships but usually the relationship is so diverse and of low magnitude that prophylactic, surgical or medical treatment is of no advantage. Racial incidence of cancer has often been used to support the argument of heredity influence but once again environment, dietary and ritualistic factors come into play, e.g. cancer of the penis is rare in Jews, where ritual circumcision is carried out, but common in Chinese, where personal hygiene is poor.

Finally, the remarkable feature of the latency of cancer between exposure to the cancer agent and the formation of the tumour will be examined. We have noted the twenty year period that follows a short exposure to certain chemicals (naphthylamines) and bladder cancer. During this period, do the changed cells lie in a suspended dormancy, until fresh stimuli potentiate the cancer, or is the progress of the cancer cell gradual, from year to year, to a final overwhelming, irreversible change? Changes detected in cervical smears may never become fully malignant, or may take five to twenty years or so to do this.

Whatever are the causes of cancer, most remain undiscovered. More work, much more work, will have to be carried out in this field of medical research, until the day when cancer becomes as controllable as bacterial infections are today. When will that day be? One dare not hazard a guess!

OBESITY

ALL FAT people have one thing in common—they 'never eat a thing'. Or at least, so they say! As Samuel Johnson said, 'If he is fat, sir, then it is plain he eats too much!' And that is the crux of the problem. Food is energy and stored energy is fat. No obese prisoners waddled out of Auswichz or Belsen where the food provided was barely able to sustain life, never enough to store as fat. The control of obesity is the control of food intake, related to energy expenditure and requirement.

Take heart, all fat persons, slimming is not beyond your capabilities. Miss Dolly Dimple, the American Fat Woman, slimmed from thirty-nine stones to eight in one year, the current world record.

Obesity is the commonest nutritional disorder in the western world, an affliction of prosperity and self-indulgence. There is no doubt that the prolonged intake of calories in excess of their expenditure, even in small daily amounts, causes obesity. However, although this is the commonest cause, it is not the only one and in certain cases genetic features are involved.

At all ages the size of the mass of adipose tissue is larger in women than in men. It represents twenty-six per cent of the weight in young women as compared to fourteen per cent in men, and as age increases the percentage rises to forty per cent in females and twenty-five per cent in males. This increase in fat, chiefly in the subcutaneous tissues, is responsible for the curvaceous outline of the woman, the mass of breast tissue, the rounded hips and thighs and the ability to sustain a bath at least five degrees hotter than any man can stand. Once the deposition has reached certain limits the aesthetic qualities are destroyed and it becomes a physical and mental hazard.

Fat is not an inert substance, however. It is constantly being broken down (catabolism) and built up (anabolism) from the carbohydrates, fats and certain amino acids (in proteins), according to the energy requirement of the body. The term adipose tissue consists of the fat cells, bulging with lipids and the supporting fibrous and cellular tissues. The deposition and mobilization of fat in adipose tissue is an active process; under favourable conditions, sugars (called glycogen, which is a complex animal 'starch' built up from simpler sugars like glucose, maltose and galactose), accumulate in the adipose tissue and are converted into fatty acids. All these metabolic activities are regulated by nervous and endocrine factors and so active is adipose tissue that it has approximately the same oxygen uptake as the lean-body (muscular) mass and its contained fluids.

Obesity is classed in two broad categories—pathological (chiefly hormonal, but perhaps genetically determined in some instances) and simple. We will deal with simple obesity.

The only effective measure in the treatment of simple obesity is the continued reduction of food intake below the energy requirements of the body. The rate at which fat is lost from the fat stores is in most cases proportional to the reduction in calorie intake. People talk blandly about calories without fully realizing what the term means. In technical terms a calorie is the amount of energy required to raise one gramme (one twenty-eighth of an ounce) through one degree centigrade. However, in medicine, the calorie described in the diet sheets is one thousand times this amount, i.e. the heat required to raise one kilogramme of water through one degree centigrade. The complete combustion of carbohydrates gives

P.P. Rubens dip.
G. Marrubini dis.
inciso nella Scuola Calamatta.

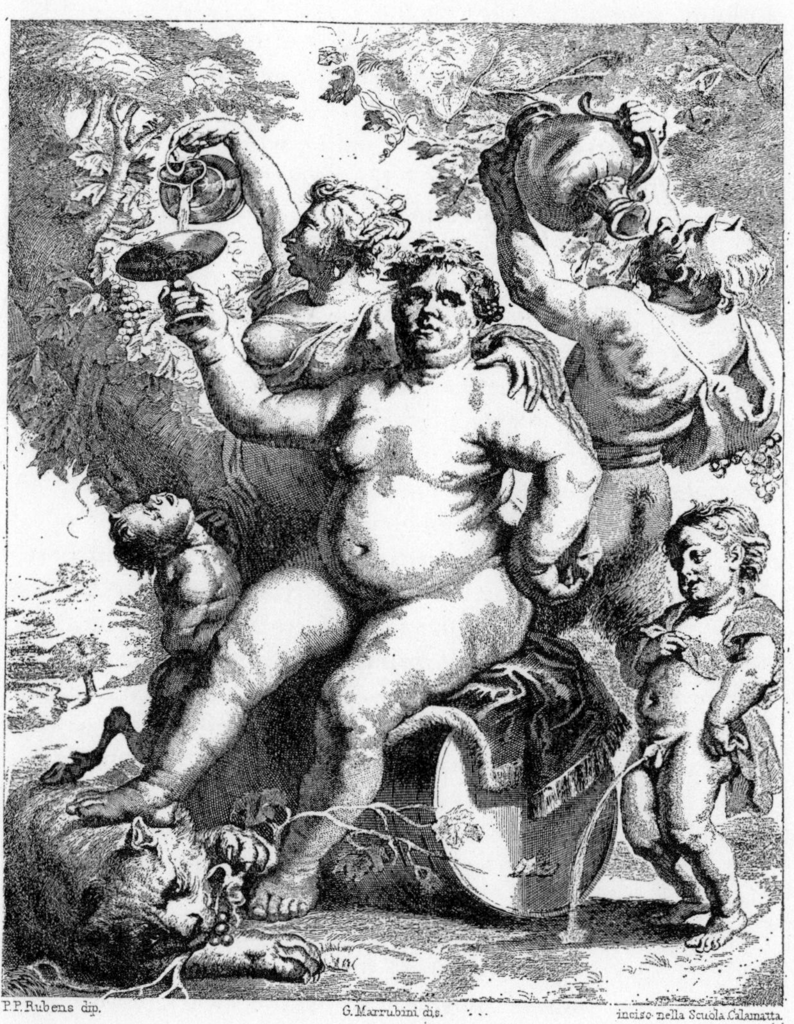

Bacchus

rise to 4·1 calories (or 4,100 conventional calories) per gramme, protein 5·4 calories per gramme and fat 9·3 calories per gramme. Thus the calorific value of fat is nearly double that of carbohydrate. The figure for protein is somewhat misleading, for body protein is oxidized incompletely, part of it being excreted as urea in the urine, which has an appreciable potential energy value. The corrected figure for protein is also 4·1 calories per gramme.

There is a great variation among foodstuffs regarding their calorific content. Apples have 36 calories per 100 grammes (3½ ozs.), carrots 22, cabbages 26, lettuce 11, tomatoes 14, oranges 33, blackcurrants 27, beans 71, bananas 74, potatoes 73, peas 61, prunes 155, raisins 236, and almonds 579. White bread has 336, brown has 250, biscuits (plain) 375, and cakes and buns 287 calories per 100 gm. Honey has 277, milk chocolate 525, plain chocolate 522, cocoa 438, jam 249 and beer 38 calories per 100 gm. Although alcohol has a calorific value of 700 cals. per 100 gm. its value as a food for energy purposes is restricted by the fact that the body can only metabolize about ten per cent per hour. Most of the foods of plant origin contain larger or smaller amounts of indigestible matter, chiefly cellulose, which is known as roughage. Man, unlike some of the ruminants and herbivores, is unable to digest this roughage, although a small quantity may be used up by the bacteria in the large intestine. The chief value of cellulose in the diet is to increase the bulk of the intestinal contents and so stimulate peristaltic movement of the bowel and combat constipation.

The main function of food is to supply energy to the animal body. This energy is required for the maintenance of body temperature, muscle movements of the heart, lungs and other organs, the performance of external work, and for the various chemical reactions, chiefly the building up of substances like proteins and hormones, in the cells. The energy requirements, consumption and expenditure usually balance in a healthy animal.

The energy output is related to oxygen consumption, since all foodstuffs are oxidized and, depending on the type of food utilized and the amount of oxygen consumed, the energy output can be calculated. Now, the expenditure of energy is related to activity but even at rest the organism requires energy to carry out all the vital processes that are occurring within it. This is called basal metabolism and if a person is kept at rest, warm and comfortable, relaxed and free from mental and physical stress under standard conditions the basal metabolism can be determined. Under these conditions the heat produced is necessary to replace that lost from the body and thus depends on surface area. The smaller the weight of an animal, the greater will be its surface area per unit of weight and hence the heat loss. Small animals like shrews and voles have to eat a fantastic amount of food per day simply to maintain a stable body temperature; their energy expenditure may be twenty to thirty times that of man. A child aged one has almost double the surface area per unit weight of a fully grown adult. For medical purposes basal metabolism is often expressed in terms of heat loss per hour, i.e. basal metabolic rate per hour or B.M.R. In certain diseases, notably thyrotoxic goitre, when the thyroid gland is overactive, the B.M.R. rises dramatically by up to forty per cent and in myxoedema, when the thyroid gland does not function adequately and the person becomes sluggish, feels the cold and has little energy, then the rate may fall by twenty or thirty per cent.

People's basal metabolic rates do vary but usually only by a small percentage. In man the basal metabolic rate is on average 40 cal/sq. metre/hour. Since the surface area of human beings is on average 1·8 sq. metres, then the basal metabolism in twenty-four hours is $40 \times 1{\cdot}8 \times 24$ hours = 1,728 calories per day.

The ingestion of food stimulates the metabolic processes in the body; a rapidly eaten meal, a thick Indian curry, promotes a feeling of flushing, warmth and sweating. This heat production is called specific dynamic action. Therefore, even under basal conditions outlined above, the amount of food eaten to produce 1,728 calories will produce additional heat loss, roughly of ten per cent (for proteins thirty per cent, fat and carbohydrates four to five per cent, on a mixed diet ten per cent). Therefore an individual has to eat 1,728 plus 173 (1,900) calories to obtain the basal number of 1,728.

What are the overall calorific requirements of man? This of course depends on the energy expenditure at work. In this context work includes relaxations and pastimes and everyday activities like washing and dressing. These simple activities usually use approximately 360 calories per day. During occupation the energy requirements may vary from writing (20 cals./hr. or 120 per six hour day), typing (180 cals./6hrs.), carpentering (840/6hrs.), light labouring (1,200), heavy labouring (1,800), coal mining (1,920), heavy blacksmithing (2,100) and wood cutting (2,400) (in 6 hours each). It is to be noted that these figures are only average. Trained persons can do work with less expenditure of energy than untrained.

Thus in twenty-four hours a clerk with a sedentary occupation needs about 2,500 calories, a housewife between 2,000 and 3,000 calories, and an average workman 3,400 calories. A blacksmith or 'heavy' workman needs 4,500 calories and a woodcutter 5,500 calories per day.

For children the calorie requirements are high relative to the body weight, for children expend a great deal of energy in growing and everyday games. Thus children of twelve to fourteen require more food than their parents.

A balanced diet per day would consist of 100 gm. of protein, 100 gm. of fat, 400 gm. of carbohydrates, giving 3,000 calories per day. In addition, essential minerals, vitamins and water are necessary. Usually two and a half litres of water are required in a temperate climate, for sedentary occupations, and at least 1·2 litres to maintain life. The quantities of vitamins and minerals needed are measured in micro- and milligrammes.

Energy expenditure, a very important consideration in the working efficiency of the body, is measured by the ratio of useful work done to the total energy available from the food consumed. In untrained subjects, doing moderate exercise, it varies between ten and twenty per cent, whereas trained subjects have levels of twenty-five per cent. However, during heavy work or prolonged hours of work, the efficiency falls off according to the duration of exercise. Most people work relatively efficiently for short periods, the length being related to the degree of training and practice.

To return to obesity, having outlined energy production and requirements, obesity and weight are not always synonymous. Heavily muscular men may be overweight but not fat, whereas individuals with poor muscular development may be of standard weight and yet at the same time be obese. The number of folds of fat that can be pinched at the waist and the overall thickness of these folds is the important criterion.

Obesity may arise at any age—during childhood, puberty and adolescence, adult life, during and after pregnancy or at the menopause. It may be sporadic, familial or a characteristic of certain races. Approximately one third of obese adults were obese in childhood. Indiscriminate overfeeding of children, especially with high calorie foods, is detrimental and a prejudice to health later in life.

Most people simply overeat because they are fond of food. The digestion of food is partly dependent upon a psychological phenomenon: thoughts of lemons promote salivation while a neatly garnished and appetizing steak initiates the outpouring of gastric juices, long before the food has entered the mouth. Indulgence of this feeling of hunger leads to excessive intake of food and so to obesity because the intake is above the calorific requirements. Sometimes, as in the case of poorer income groups, too much cheap carbohydrate material is eaten. The number of excess calories consumed each day may be quite small but it has been reported that only an extra nine calories per day will give rise to a weight gain of one gram of fat per day which over a period of twenty years amounts to fifteen pounds.

Alcohol, as I have already mentioned (p. 47) is highly calorific. One pint of beer contains 180 calories, one glass of brandy 73, one of whisky 90, white wine 100, rum 65, sherry 53, port 86, cider 110 and champagne 60. So what might be termed a delicate evening snack of two pints of beer (360), one whisky (90), one chow mein (400), a doughnut, two mince pies (1,066) and a cup of tea (6) or coffee (6) equals 1,922 calories, or almost the total basal expenditure of a person per day. If he eats another two muffins (270) and one piece of fruit cake (320), he can shut up shop for the remaining twenty-three and a half hours left in the day, providing he has a sedentary occupation.

Compare this with the following: four cups of tea (24 cals.), one apple (60), one grapefruit (24), one portion of cabbage (8) and one of carrot (15), boiled potatoes (4 oz. equals 88 cals.), two energen rolls (36), ryvita (two pieces equals 68 cals.), cottage cheese (45 cals. per 1½ oz.), one boiled egg (92), one yoghurt (95), lean rump roasted (2 oz. equals 142 cals.), chicken (2 oz. equals 112), ham (2 oz. equals 124), steamed haddock (3 oz. equals 84), lobster (3 oz. equals 70) and lettuce (6 oz. equals 18): a grand total of 1105 calories (or 2¾ doughnuts).

Some people find that they put on weight after stopping smoking. This is simply due to the overeating of sweets or foodstuffs. The indiscriminate nibbling of food between meals can lead to a considerable calorific intake; fruit and unsweetened beverages are much preferable.

Physical activity is important in the regulation of weight but over-emphasis on this fact alone is wrong. The correct way to lose weight is to diet. For example, a five mile walk will cause the expenditure of three hundred calories, which is the equivalent of two slices of bread and butter, one and a half pints of beer or one mince pie. The exercise necessary for the combustion of one pound of fat amounts to walking nearly seventy miles, or running forty-three miles. Thus the average person who is one and a half stones overweight has to walk one thousand, four hundred and seventy miles without food to achieve his required weight loss. If an individual's physical activity is high but he continually exceeds his calorific intake, then obesity will result. When a person changes from an occupation involving a good deal of physical activity to one of a sedentary nature, or goes by car instead of taking the morning and evening walk to the bus, he should immediately reduce his calorie intake. Once obesity is established the amount of exercise taken becomes more and more reduced with a further resulting increase in the obese state.

Psychological disturbances may be a factor in obesity. Some people consume more food when nervous or worried and obesity is well known to develop rapidly after a sudden and severe emotional upset. However, boredom, loneliness, anxiety, depression, tension and frustration are only the root cause. The increase of adipose tissue is still related to food intake. Cut this down and the amount of fat will decrease.

Some people, although not hungry, experience an irresistible desire to eat. They are compulsive eaters. Others nibble at night—the 'night-eaters'. These people may have underlying alterations in gastric mobility, blood sugar levels and nervous control in the satiety centres of the brain, compared with normal subjects.

However, there is no doubt that some people maintain a high quantity of adipose tissue despite great variations in calorific control. Some people have a constant weight over many years despite excessive food intake, while others respond immediately to a slight increase in calorific consumption by an upsurge in weight.

Having excluded the obvious pathological types of obesity due to hormonal disturbances, which regress with the correct treatment of the underlying conditions, one must conclude that certain obese persons have a degree of adipose tissue which simply underlies either a facilitated absorption from the bowel (transported to the fat deposits) or an increased conversion of sugars into fat, with perhaps a deficient release of sugars from fats when the occasion demands. There is no doubt that obesity runs in families, for up to half of the offspring are obese when one of the parents is fat and up to two thirds when both are obese. Eighty per cent of fat children have at least one obese parent but only nine per cent of children of normal parents are overweight. It is difficult to determine whether familial obesity is due to a genetic abnormality or simply due to environmental factors.

The distribution of the fat in simple obesity is generalized, affecting the face, trunk and limbs. When obesity is gross, large deposits of fat hang from the upper arms, the breasts are huge and pendulous, drooping down over the anterior abdominal walls; a fat apron descends from the anterior abdominal wall over the pubic region on to the thighs and rolls of fat envelop the waist, buttocks and hips and the normal contour of the legs is obliterated by deposits round the thighs, knees and ankles. Locomotion becomes difficult.

Excessive sweating can lead to skin infection in the axillae (armpits), groin and under the breasts. The skin tends to become more coarse than normal and there may be excessive growth of the hair, especially on the face and pubic region. Menstrual irregularities are common in obese women. The blood pressure is often normal but many patients complain of tiredness, lack of energy and shortness of breath on exertion due to their increased bulk and possible fatty infiltration into the heart. Obese patients are liable to psychological disurbances, including a sense of inferiority, social exclusion and ridicule and also anxiety/depressive states. A number of patients with severe obesity become mentally sluggish but there are notable exceptions, e.g. Samuel Johnson.

One of the problems associated with pregnancy is maternal obesity. Before its onset many of these women are of normal weight but the majority who develop this type of obesity are overweight before conception. However, women who are obese before pregnancy may not increase in size during it and, on the other hand, being underweight is no guarantee that maternal obesity will not occur. The onset may be rapid, usually between the third and sixth month. If it arises after pregnancy, during lactation, the onset may be delayed two to three months. Some people unfortunately gain weight with each pregnancy, usually remaining stationary during the intervening periods. Doctors now know that a weight gain of more than one pound per week during the middle and later trimesters of pregnancy is unfavourable for the mother and child. There is often very little tendency to spontaneous reduction in weight once the pregnancy is concluded. Women with maternal obesity produce an excess of large babies. The cause for this rapid gain in weight is unknown. Many of these patients feel hungry all the time, others find that carbohydrates control nausea, some cheerfully 'eat for two' and with some the reduction in energy expenditure by giving up work and exercise, plus boredom, leads to this excessive conversion of food to fat.

There are many hazards of obesity and it definitely reduces the normal expectation of life. Disorders of the heart and circulation are common, so are gallstones and gall bladder trouble. Appendicitis incidence is double the normal and they suffer more commonly from flat feet, osteoarthritis of the spine, hip and knee, hernias of all description, of which hiatus hernia (when part of the stomach is pushed through the small opening of the oesophagus into the chest) is the most common, acute and chronic bronchitis, pneumonia, cirrhosis of the liver, diabetes mellitus, gout and certain forms of cancer.

But what of the treatment of obesity? The only effective measure in the control of simple obesity is the continued reduction of food intake below energy expenditure. If, after going on a diet, your weight at first reduces and then levels out again, then a further reduction of food is necessary. Tablets and other slimming aids are grossly subsidiary to this reduction in calorie intake. The rate of loss of weight is proportional to the deficiency of food. The degree of improvement depends on the attitude and co-operation of the persons concerned, bearing in mind that there is no short cut to success. Simply stick to a rigid diet and increase the amount of exercise. Many slimming foods are false economy because they still contain a substantial level of carbohydrates.

There are many diets but the most important feature is the strict adherence to a low calorie intake. One thousand and one thousand five hundred calorie diets are the most popular but in severe cases three hundred and even zero calorie diets have been used in hospital. Turkish baths simply cause loss of salt and water which is rapidly put back by the long cool drink afterwards. Fat massage-vibrators give a feeling of wellbeing and little else.

Because of their low calorie value a fairly liberal intake of fresh fruit, green vegetables and salads is allowed but cut out bananas, peas, grapes, etc. Saccharine can be used for sweetening. There should always be an adequate intake of minerals, vitamins and proteins.

When the desired weight has been reached then a strict watch should be kept on any weight increase for if a person lapses into previous eating habits obesity returns. Obesity is a problem that can only be controlled with perseverance, decreased food intake and an optimistic attitude.

Obesity has always been with us but, whereas nowadays obese people are regarded usually with a mixture of pity and disgust, in previous centuries excessive fat folk were regarded by their fellows as persons worthy of admiration and awe. The paviors of Cambridge used to say, 'God bless you, sir!' to a huge professor when he walked over their work. Fatness has also been the butt of good-natured jocularity. The following lines were inscribed on the tomb of a corpulent chandler:

Here lies in earth an honest fellow,
Who died by fat and lived by tallow.

One of the most prodigious specimens of obesity was Daniel

Lambert, whose remains lie in the burial ground of St. Martin's, Stamford Baron, covered by a black slate, inscribed as follows:

Altus in animo, in Corpore Maximus.
In remembrance of that prodigy in nature,
Daniel Lambert, a native of Leicester, who was possessed
of an exalted and convivial mind;
and, in personal greatness, had no competitor;
he measured 3 ft. 1 in. round the leg,
9 ft. 4 in. round the body,
and weighed 52 st. 11 lb.!
He departed this life on the 21st June, 1809,
aged 39 years.
As a mark of respect, this
stone is erected by his friends in Leicester.

It was not until the spring of 1806 that Lambert overcame his repugnance to publicly exhibiting himself. After that period he resided nearly five months in the metropolis, and then travelled about the country, gratifying the curiosity of his countrymen, until the time of his death. He had apparently for some time shown symptoms of dropsy but otherwise had had no sickness to indicate the suddenness of his death. Two suits of Lambert's clothes were preserved at the Wagon and Horses Inn, in St. Martin's, Stamford. Seven men of average size could be enclosed within his waistcoat, without apparently breaking a stitch. His coffin measured six feet four inches long, four feet four inches wide, two feet four inches deep and contained one hundred and twelve superficial feet of elm. It was built on two axletrees and four wheels, upon which his remains were drawn to their place of interment. His grave was dug with a gradual sloping for many yards and about twenty men were employed for nearly half an hour in getting the huge corpse to its last abode. Mr. Lambert was a great sportsman in his early life, according to the records, his bulk not having increased much above the ordinary size until he was about twenty-one or twenty-two years old. He ate moderately and never drank anything but water.

Obesity therefore, one of the medical problems of today, has gained for one man, at least, a place in the annals of history.

Dr. Hunter, in his 'Culina', gives the receipt for an omelette the invention of a lady, who had it regularly served at her table, three days in a week, and who died at the age of ninety-seven, with a piece of it in her mouth. The doctor adds that, in consequence of this accidental longevity, eggs rose ninety per cent in the small town of Wells, in North America, where the old lady was born and died.

Timbs: *Doctors and Patients*, 1873.

A bit in the morning is better than nothing all day.
An apple, an egg, and a nut, you may eat after a slut.
After dinner sit awhile, after supper walk a mile.
Who goes to bed supperless, all night tumbles and tosses.
Cheese is a peevish elf, it digests all but itself.

Eighteenth-century poem.

TRANSPLANTATION

THE LAST decade of medicine will always be recalled as the age of transplantation. With the advent of heart transplantation public interest in, and outcry against medical techniques reached new levels. Suddenly everyone was concerned. Volumes were written in the press and spoken on television, and such was the sensational aspect that ill-taste, poor judgement and ill-considered remarks abounded. Mistrust over the criteria of death sprang up in the public's mind, a public that had for years trusted the medical profession's opinion on this aspect. Distinguished people in medicine not only openly stated that many medical correspondents were singularly ignorant and mischievous but had inadvertently caused the death of patients waiting for potential organ donors whose relatives had lately refused consent due to the adverse publicity given to the whole subject of organ transplantation.

The concept of death and the necessity for the immediate removal of organs, still viable, were the criteria at the root of the problem. Naturally the public, to whom death is an unknown and therefore awesome factor, were alarmed that vital tissues were taken from a patient before death had been irrevocably determined and this fear was even more marked in the case of heart transplantation as the heart has a particular emotional connotation as being the 'seat' of life. However, the heart can continue to pump in a dead person, in a guillotined man or a person who has been hanged, for example, and the maintenance of pulsation can be continued for hours or even days if a heart-lung machine is used. Therefore in many countries, for example the U.S.A. and France, the concept of brain death has been instituted. If, after a searching examination by medical specialists, a variety of criteria has been satisfied, the patient is pronounced dead and vital organs can be removed for transplantation. In this country, fear of the possibility of human error, however diligent and stringent the examination, however independent the medical specialists, is foremost in the public's mind.

The way round these dilemmas is to allow people to contract in or out of transplantation (perhaps the latter course is the easier of the two). A simple tattoo or card could be supplied to those persons not wishing to participate in transplantation. More detailed information and co-operation could be given to the press, in an effort to produce better relations and to reduce sensationalism and misrepresentation. Transplantation has a dynamic part to play in medical progress; almost three thousand young people die per year from kidney diseases alone, many of whom could be kept alive with transplants. Heart, liver, lung, larynx and eyes have all been utilized in transplantation. Cornea, blood, arteries, cartilage and bone have all been obtained from the dead and used in the living.

But to return to the subject—the transplantation of tissues is the replacement of accidentally damaged or destroyed tissues, the destruction usually being caused by disease. For the graft to serve any useful purpose the cells must survive and function normally. Tissues from the same person transferred from one region to another, for example, pieces of skin taken from the leg and transferred to the arm, will quickly be incorporated in their new situation and will multiply. Tissues transferred from one identical twin to another will also have a successful outcome—many kidney transplants have now survived ten years with perfect function. It is only when tissues are transferred from one individual to another, or between animal species, that rejection occurs. The whole problem of transplantation is tissue rejection. This is the barrier that has to be overcome.

But what are the causes of this phenomenon? Animals must have a germ-free internal environment. The skin contains millions of bacteria, many of which produce minute amounts of acids that prevent disease-inducing (or pathogenic) bacteria and fungi from settling and multiplying there. Similarly, the bowel, especially the large intestine, is crammed with bacteria that provide vitamins in return for the nourishment they obtain from undigested food. These are the two surfaces of an animal, the internal and the external, representing a cylindrical form. Between these surfaces, however, there exists a germ-free area where the cells function in a sterile environment. The invasion of bacteria or viruses into this area produces an infectious disease. Since these pathogenic organisms are continually trying to invade the body, a large, highly mobile army of cells lies in readiness. These are the white blood corpuscles and they are reinforced by reserves from the bone marrow, lymph nodes, liver and other organs. Once bacteria invade, the white cells literally gobble them up but if the poisons produced by these germs are effective, or if the number of germs is proportionately large or the white cells are depleted for any reason, then the battle swings in favour of the pathogenic organisms and fever, general ill-health, rashes and abscesses, etc., ensue. The body is still not beaten, however. The special fighting cells of the lymph nodes, liver and other organs rapidly form antibodies, taking between five to ten days to do so and these antibodies pour out into the blood to neutralize the invading germs. Thus, in the pre-antibiotic area, the crises of pneumonia occurred when the temperature suddenly fell with the out-pouring of antibodies, if the patient was going to recover. The body is ready for an invasion at any time, and procedures like vaccination and immunisation (as against tetanus) simply supply the information to these special cells to prepare them for future needs. Once the cells have become conditioned to an organism a state of immunity exists.

In transplantation a foreign material is placed in the body. Each tissue consists of proteins. Each protein has a distinct and unique structure for the individual and is only duplicated in identical twins. When the 'foreign' material, be it a heart, kidney or liver, has been in the receiver's body for a few hours, the white cells have already begun to mobilize to destroy what they believe to be an invading organism. Within two to three days round, plump cells (lymphocytes) are invading the transplant and the rejection process begins. Antibodies to neutralize and destroy the foreign proteins (antigens) are formed by the special cells outlined above and after five to ten days in the case of skin the graft is converted into a necrotic scab and ceases to function. The same rejection process is common to all tissues. However, in the case of corneal grafts (the cornea being the clear, bulging area on the front of the eye) where there are no blood vessels concerned, the destroying cells, normally transported by the blood stream, cannot reach the graft, and it survives permanently.

The same biological phenomenon takes place throughout all higher vertebrates; goldfish reject foreign grafts no less vigorously than men, chickens or rabbits.

What can be done to prevent rejection? Firstly, all the white cells in the body can be destroyed by either drugs or X-rays and the graft will then survive indefinitely. Since, however, bacteria will also be given a free hand under these conditions, the animal must be nursed under germ-free conditions. In present-day transplantation techniques enough of the drugs are given to the recipient to lower his white cell count so that only slow rejection of the graft takes place, but not enough to impair his ability to combat infection. This is a delicate dividing line and requires regular supervision by medical experts. New drugs will be developed in this field as the problems of rejection become clearer. Secondly, tissues can be taken that closely resemble the recipient's, those of an identical twin being ideal and in other instances those of near relations such as brothers or fathers, etc., are employed.

Finally, a vaccine may be prepared in the future which, when injected into a developing foetus in the womb, will enable grafts to be performed successfully. For the developing baby grows so quickly initially that it is unable to recognize its own tissues and passes through a stage when any cells given to it are accepted as its own. This is the state of chimerism, first identified in unidentical twin calves whose placentas touched and passed very small amounts of blood from one to another, so that the calves were found to have mixed blood groups and each would accept blood from its 'twin' with impunity.

There are many problems remaining in transplantation but it has now become an established part of surgery and medicine, offering hope and a new life to those who suffer from conditions which were once beyond the realm of cure.

In a sense, mammals have been constantly exposed to grafts since they evolved—by Nature herself—during pregnancy. Every foetus is a graft and possesses, even at an early stage, antigens inherited from its father that may be lacking in its mother. The biological success of mammals is strong evidence that dispensations apply. The complete vascular quarantine of the foetus is probably the basis of its exemption from immunological rejections.

Billingham, 1962

SLUMS

SLUMS, a word that conjures up a world of dim lights, cold rooms, orange box cribs, scabies and suffering; a twilight existence for thousands of children, ill-fed, ill-shod and unwanted; a breeding ground for human vermin, the social misfits, the perverted and the mentally sick; generations nurtured by insecurity, strains and tensions that twist and warp the mind, leaving distorted social impressions that last for life; a horror of human suffering translated into mental strife. To comprehend the physical suffering is easy, the mental anguish impossible.

There are nearly twenty thousand men, women and children effectively homeless in the British Isles. They live in local or governmental hostels with little privacy. Another 1,800,000 houses are officially condemned as 'unfit for human habitation'.

As Shelter declares, the home should meet two criteria: it should be a place where individuals and families can be themselves for better or worse, can obtain peace and security and can flourish both mentally and physically. Secondly, it should be an effective base for daily life, providing rest and relaxation and again the mental strength for participation in our highly pressurized and competitive society. Families nagged by insecurity, over-crowded so that they live with constant strain and tension, lacking any kind of privacy, surrounded by dampness and infestation that spread disease, living in physical danger because of the dilapidated condition of the property and cheated of the essential facilities that others take for granted are, in our view, homeless.

Conditions such as these are a breeding ground for mental illnesses. The prevalence of schizophrenia in the east end of London, among the slums, is twice the national average and depression is more common by fifty per cent.

Let us examine both types of patients. The majority of the depressed persons are females between twenty-five and thirty-five, who present with hysteria, agitation, tearfulness and aggression. They tend to veer away from contraception, either through ignorance, religion or atavistic submission to the male and the possible solace of a child which, according to one report, is necessary to fill the void in a humdrum existence concerned with survival. Only during psychotic episodes do they show hostility towards their husbands or lovers regarding sex. Unfortunately the males are rarely able to provide their wives with any degree of social support when confronted by adverse or impossible housing conditions. Slums in fact breed a mental separation between husbands and wives, leading to inadequacies, frustration and aggression. Self-esteem becomes non-existent, the depressed patient drifts despairingly, burdened with a large family, poor income and distorted environment.

Any economically depressed area becomes the precipitating ground for schizophrenics who wander in from the surrounding parts as they slide down the social scale, impelled on their downward path by the social inadequacy resulting from their mental abnormalities. Often they bring their fairly normal hard-working families with them. In such surroundings they are liable to further and repeated breakdowns and often the tenuous family ties become broken, leaving the schizophrenic alone in an environment indifferent to him and his problems.

Some slums have improved very little since the era of Bob Cratchit and Tiny Tim, although, as in Dickens' famous novel, families with good, stable relationships, free from mental stress, can survive poverty unscathed. However, should mental illness, physical incapacity, husband (or wife) desertion or a family bereavement further reduce the income and thus aggravate an already critical situation, then the home becomes broken and the children shuttled about in a transitional world of home and homes.

Slums are therefore more than bricks and mortar, hot and cold, indoor toilets; they are a problem of education, hygiene, rehousing and social pride and while they still exist they remain as monuments to human suffering, both physical and mental.

APPENDICITIS—IN RETROSPECT

IN 1837 Burne, a physician at the Westminster Hospital, called attention to the following case: 'Walking one afternoon with a medical friend, he requested me to call and see a case of a very obscure nature under the care of himself and a hospital physician, which he feared was going on to a fatal termination. The patient, a baronet's coachman, fifty-seven years of age, had become affected three weeks previously with febrile movement, succeeded by vomiting and constipation, which required the use of the strongest cathartics to procure dejections. In the course of the second week he complained of pain in the ilio-inguinal region, for which leeches and a blister had been applied; and about this period there occurred also retention of urine.

When I examined him, he was lying on his back in bed, much exhausted, with the tongue beginning to get brown and dry and the pulse frequent and weak. He vomited frequently and the bowels were so obstinate that no aperient but croton oil would act upon them. He still laboured under retention of urine, the belly was full and tense, and in examining the region of the caecum, to which he referred as the seat of pain, I discovered immediately a circumscribed, hard, deep-seated tumour, the size of a small orange and gave it as my opinion that the disease was situated in the caecum or appendix. After this he survived not more than eight days, the vomiting, obstinate constipation, pain and retention of urine having continued to the last. The post mortem revealed an abscess of the appendix.'

Today appendicitis is one of the commonest abdominal emergencies, and very rarely associated with death. But it is definitely a disease of the twentieth century, being rare in India, and also in Africa. It has been found in a mummy of a young royal princess of Egypt, described in Coptic jars as the 'worm of the bowel'. For the appendix, lying at the commencement of the large bowel (caecum region) in the right lower region of the abdomen, closely resembles in size the common earth worm, and for years was known as the vermiform appendix.

One of the first recorded cases of inflammation of this organ was by Mestivier in 1759. His patient was a man of forty-five who developed pain and an abscess in the right side, which the physician incised and evacuated a pint or so of pus. The patient died and at post mortem he found a large pin, very rusty and so corroded in certain places that 'the least touch would have broken it'.

Other famous physicians like Thomas Addison (of Addison's disease and anaemia fame) and Richard Bright (of Bright's disease) both recognized that the appendix could be the site of inflammation. This was in 1839 but most doctors continued to ignore the appendix as a cause of disease and concentrated on the small and large bowel for pathology, and almost all patients continued to die from perforation and peritonitis.

Ten years later Hancock, a surgeon at Charing Cross Hospital, received a delicate woman of about seven and a half months pregnant into his wards, suffering from severe abdominal pain. On the seventh day she delivered of a small baby that died, and by the tenth the pain was acute with a hard swelling appearing on the right side. Six leeches were applied, and warm fomentations and calomel given. By the seventeenth day she was in extremis and under chloroform (anaesthesia had just been instituted) the large abscess was incised. Two weeks after the operation she discharged several small concretions which 'from their size', said Hancock have been impacted in and escaped from the appendix vermiformis. The patient recovered and was later sent home quite well.

An American, Fitz, of Philadelphia, used the term appendicitis (to mean inflammation of the appendix) and suggested its removal. Krönlein in the same year (1886) reported the first surgical removal of the appendix, but the patient died. In 1888 Sir Frederick Treves put forward the view that the removal of the appendix might safeguard against the spread of inflammation.

On 14th June, 1902, it was noted, 'The King is rather ill with severe chill. Unable to dine'. Sir Francis Laking diagnosed appendicitis, and although peritonitis was developing quickly, the doctor decided that it would be wrong to alarm the King who was exceedingly irritable and depressed and who told him, 'If this goes on, I shall give it all up. I shall abdicate.' He was put on a milk diet, and was told to rest in bed. In this way it was hoped to avoid postponement of the coronation at Westminster on 26th June.

On 23rd June Sir Thomas Barlow and Sir Francis Laking informed the King that he would certainly die unless an operation was performed without delay. King Edward VII argued furiously with the doctors before exclaiming, 'Laking, I will stand no more of this. Leave the room at once.' Pleading his continued devotion to his royal patient, Laking brought in Lord Lister and Sir Thomas Smith. Lister was dubious. Smith agreed that Treves should carry out the operation. At 12.25 p.m. Treves began the incision on the abdomen (whose girth was forty-eight inches) and during the ensuing forty minutes the appendix was removed. Magnus (1964) reports: 'In the streets of the capital the news reverberated like a thunderclap and a dress rehearsal of the coronation in Westminster Abbey was transformed into an impromptu service of intercession.' Appendicitis had become a fashionable disease.

In spite of appendicitis being so common today, very little is known of the underlying cause. It affects persons of highly civilized countries (such as Europeans, Australasians and Americans) but should persons from areas where it is rare move into these countries, then they acquire the local susceptibility to the disease. It is also commonest in the professional and managerial class and it has been observed that among those who do not get the disease the diet is much simpler, contains a larger relative bulk of coarse vegetables and other cellulose-containing foodstuffs, and perhaps a smaller constituent of meat. The role of diet, tinned foods, toxic chemicals in causing appendicitis is unknown, even today.

In many ways appendicitis still remains as mysterious as when John Parkinson first described it in 1812; the Egyptian 'worm of the bowel' still wriggles.

THE FATE OF THE JAVAN RHINO

THERE ARE fewer than thirty Javan rhino in the world today. All are to be found in the three hundred square mile Udjung Kulon Nature Reserve in western Java and their situation is critical.

There are four thousand million people in the world today; By the year 2000 this will have risen, according to calculations, to 6,270,000,000. Will there ever be fewer than thirty again? According to Professor Ehrlich of California: 'If I were a gambler, I would take even money that England will not exist in the year 2000, and give ten to one that the life of the average Briton will be of a lower quality than it is today.' He contends that Britain, like Japan, is one of a number of overdeveloped countries, poor in resources and too large in population, which, if present trends continue, will be a small group of impoverished islands containing at least seventy million hungry people. It has also been estimated that in the next four hundred years man will stand ten to the square yard throughout the world.

The population of the world did not pass the one hundred million mark until after the time of the old Kingdom of Egypt, and did not exceed five hundred million until the mid-seventeenth century. It reached a thousand million in the mid-nineteenth century and two thousand million in 1930. Thus the world population doubled in the two hundred years between 1650 and 1850 and doubled again in the next hundred years. It is predicted that the population will have doubled again by 1980, that is, in the short space of thirty years. The number of 'hatches' per day is 270,000 and the number of 'despatches' 143,000, an excess of 128,000 births or approximately fifty million new inhabitants of the globe per year. Technologically underdeveloped regions have a higher than average birth rate; the proverbial Chinaman born every third second, the one million new Indian faces per month, these are realities. In the decade 1951-1961 the population of India rose by twenty-two per cent, with a population density of 370 per square mile over its 3,768,100 square miles of territory, a grand total of 735 million. In India alone only forty per cent of the land is available for cultivation, mainly in the valley of the Ganges. The annual production of less than twenty million tons of rice is completely inadequate to feed the population and the people are grossly protein-deficient. Because of religious beliefs cattle are seldom killed and yield very little milk. India only survives with foreign aid from the major food producers and soaks up the surplus corn and other foodstuffs at an alarming rate. The populations of America and Canada also continue to expand. 5·3 million people lived in the three million square miles (an area as large as Europe) of the United States in the year 1800; by 1900 this had increased to seventy-six million and by 1965 to over one hundred and eighty-five million, a density of sixty-two persons per square mile. In the year 1800 3·7 million lived in Canada with an area of four million square miles; by 1900 5·4 million and by 1965 nineteen million. The present population of Britain is fifty-two million and this should reach eighty million by the year 2000 if the present birth trends continue. Recently the population problem has been exaggerated and made increasingly complex by the immigration from the Commonwealth, particularly from the Caribbean lands. Thirty-seven thousand coloured immigrants entered Britain in 1966, resulting in an established coloured population of a million people in Britain over the last decade. During the period 1950 to 1960 the increase in population in the United Kingdom was somewhat masked by the emigration to Australia, Canada etc. with a net loss of seventy thousand in 1953 and fifteen thousand in 1956-57. But a positive influx was established in 1958 by the increase in immigrants. In the year 1800 only nine million inhabitants occupied England and Wales with two million in Scotland. In 1900 the figures were thirty-two and a half million and four and a half million, in 1965 forty-seven million and five million respectively. The density of population per square mile has risen in England and Wales from 152 in 1800 to 558 in 1900 and 860 in 1969, while in Scotland it has risen from 60 (1800) to 150 (1900) to 180 (1969).

At the present time, therefore, England has become one of the world's most overcrowded countries; eighty per cent of the population crush into cities that spread and sprawl across the countryside, gobbling up precious land at the rate of a county the size of Cambridgeshire every seven years, poisoning the rivers, polluting the atmosphere and exterminating the wild life. The greater the expansion of human population, the more wild-life diminishes.

For over sixty-five million years, to the time of the Cretaceous period, man has evolved from the lower primates that still exist today in Prosimian group (lower primates) of the tree shrews, lemurs, bush babies and tarsiers, through the higher primates (anthropoidean group of Old and New World monkeys) and past the anthropoid apes—the gibbon, orang-utan, chimpanzee and gorilla, our nearest relatives. During the mid-pleistocene period, five hundred thousand years ago, changes in brain size and function, upright stance and delicate finger movements began to evolve, culminating, during the last ten thousand years, in modern man as we now know him. From the manipulative dexterity of his fingers and hands and the inventive capacity of his expanding intellectual functions, the modern technological age has derived. What are the consequences?

Half of the woodland, perhaps thirty to forty million square miles, has been destroyed, nowhere more noticeably than in

England where vast forests once abounded until the Middle Ages. With the removal of trees, the exposed surface layers of the soil are frequently moved by the physical agencies of wind and rain, erosion ensues and fertile plains, made barren and lifeless, form vast dustpans that now exist in many areas of the United States.

Man also deposits waste on the earth's surface; some, like the biological waste of decomposing bodies and excretory materials, are utilized by bacteria and other lower animals and are reincorporated in the biological cycle. Some, like the wastes of industrial processes and domestic origin can never be utilized. Radioactive materials from nuclear reactors present additional hazards for leakage into the seas or atmosphere could lead to a generalized pollution which would not only have immediate effects, like cancer induction, but would cause harm to future generations through alteration of the hereditary genes. Britain now has eight nuclear reactors, situated close to the coasts so that they can obtain the enormous quantities of water for cooling purposes, and leakage of materials from the uranium fission process, like strontium and caesium, which are taken up by the tissues, especially by the bones, could have a disastrous effect on mankind. Already strontium ninety has been incorporated from the atmosphere (following nuclear tests) by rainfall and from the lichens of the Arctic and the mosses and grasses of the countryside proceeds thence to the bones, flesh and milk of grazing animals. Children in America and Europe now have seven times the amount of radioactive strontium ninety in their bones than that of previous generations. The level at which these substances become dangerous is not known. At present radioactive solid wastes are packed into special containers and dumped into the sea, some of the more lethal being stored pending final disposal.

The recent death of thousands of sea birds from oil pollution in the *Torrey Canyon* disaster pinpoints another man-made disaster. Four hundred and fifty million tons of oil pass British waters annually and the indiscriminate dumping of small amounts by coastal vessels has led to a serious increase in pollution. The spillage of oil is thought to be in the order of thirty thousand tons annually, in this country alone. The cost to marine and bird life is incalculable at the present time and is increasing in magnitude annually.

The death of thousands of fish in the recent Rhine disaster, when poisonous chemicals were inadvertently released, emphasizes the problems of river pollution. In Britain, a land of beautiful, fast-flowing rivers, nothing is sadder than to witness the demise of a fresh water stream, abounding with fish, and the formation in its place of a dense, dark-coloured, polluted sewer, devoid of all forms of life. Poison chemicals continue to pour directly into the rivers, or indirectly through seepage from the land where they have been employed as pesticides. Oils and detergents are washed into the river from roads, workshops and garages. Sewage effluents discharge continually into the major rivers, ton upon ton of excretia per day. The effects of pollutants on rivers are as follows: (a) reduction in oxygen necessary to support life, (b) an increase in temperature from water returned from cooling processes—about fifteen million gallons per day, and (c) the addition of poisons, oil films and insoluble particulate matter which has a direct effect on animal and plant metabolism. Work has commenced on cleaning our rivers but the demands from an increasing population and the associated industrial processes will continue to pollute the waters for generations to come, if not for all time.

The problem of poisons supplied to the land has repercussions far beyond the direct effect it has on wildlife. The whole ecology of an area becomes upset. Synthetic pesticides have now been in increasing use for twenty-five years. The most dangerous are the organochlorines. The mass deaths of birds in 1960 and 1961 led to a voluntary ban of the use on spring sown wheat of aldrin and dieldrin, two of the most poisonous organochlorines. After the report of the 1964

Advisory Committee of Pesticides the voluntary restrictions were then extended and their use in chemicals for the garden and sheep dips ended. No restriction was placed on D.D.T. In 1964 the decline in predatory birds was observed, but four years were to elapse before the precise mechanism was elucidated. These substances affect certain hormones which regulate the mobilization of calcium, so leading to excessive egg breakage, mainly in hawks. Hungary, Sweden and Denmark have now banned D.D.T. but a hundred and nineteen million pounds of aldrin were produced in the U.S.A. in 1964-65 and a hundred and forty-one million pounds of D.D.T. Residues of these long-lived chemicals have been found in most living creatures, including man, from the Antarctic to the far north of Canada. As L. F. Stickel concludes in her recent report 'the impact of these new components on the eco-system appears as death, reproductive impairment, disruption of species balance, and behavioural alteration'. Thus the chemicals on the grasses enter the bodies of insects, birds and small animals which depend on the grasses for food and so ultimately to the bird carnivores, especially the eagles, hawks and falcons.

Nearly two and a half million tons of smoke pollutants are delivered to the atmosphere annually, an unappetizing confluence of black soot, tar, ash, sulphur dioxide and acid, which rains down upon us continually, choking the lungs and fine air passages, causing us to wheeze, spit and eventually die from respiratory failure. Add twenty-four million tons of carbon monoxide, and fifty-two million tons of sulphuric acid and one has a destructive process that causes ten million pounds worth of damage to agriculture annually and indirectly fifty thousand deaths. The famous London smog of 1952 killed four thousand people and many prize cattle at the Smithfield Show in just a few days. The advent of the Clean Air Act, long overdue and still not adequately enforced in many areas, should ensure that such catastrophes are a thing of the past (in the London area alone the smoke pollution has dropped by seventy per cent in the last fifteen years). Exhaust fumes from cars, however, provide yet another atmospheric hazard. The now famous Los Angeles smog, occurring for about one fifth of the year, is due to the five million gallons of petrol burnt every day. The same problem will become manifest in Britain unless our government follows the lead of the United States and insists on car modifications so that only a low level of exhaust fumes is permitted to enter the atmosphere.

We choke, poison and pollute our resources, breed, save lives and live longer, crowd and crush into all available living space. Wildlife is the first to suffer under these conditions. 'You may say that the extinction of species has been going on since the dawn of life; after all we have no dinosaurs with us today. But man, it seems, has accelerated the extinction rate of species in some animal groups by a factor of four. This has meant that more than one vertebrate animal form has become extinct per year during my lifetime. In the U.S.A. alone, eight kinds of fish are believed to have become extinct since the end of the Second World War. What happened to the passenger-pigeon and the Carolina parakeet is still happening in this day and age. Many people say that man, the most dangerous predatory animal in the world, is just operating the laws of evolution and this is no doubt true, but the point is that man is the first predator to realize what he is doing. I think it was Mark Twain that said "Man is the only animal that blushes or needs to".' (Peter Scott, 1967.)

The Survival Service Commission of the International Union for the Conservation of Nature publishes a Red Book of Endangered Species. At this moment no less than eight hundred and seventeen species of mammals and birds are threatened with extinction. Here are a few: out of the seven recognized species of tiger, six of them are endangered, perhaps twelve Javan tigers exist, sixty Caspian, a hundred and fifty Siberian, but the Bali, Chinese and Sumatran tigers may be extinct. The Dibatag, an elegant deer in Ethiopia and Somalia, now numbers less than two thousand; the Asian lion now exists precariously in only one small area of some four hundred and eighty square miles of the Gir Forest in India, relentless hunting by British military personnel in the nineteenth century having reduced the numbers to the point of extinction. There were only one hundred remaining in 1900 but the number has now increased to almost three hundred. The rare wild Bactrian camel was assumed to be extinct but recent expeditions by Chinese and Mongolian zoologists have confirmed the existence of a few remaining animals. The Tasmanian wolf, a carnivorous marsupial, is also almost extinct, due to unrestricted hunting and the introduction of the Dingo on to the Australian mainland. The onyx and giant sable antelope have only been saved by rigorous protection and preservation of habitat; while the gorilla and orang-utan, our close relatives, continue to diminish alarmingly, chiefly due to the destruction of their habitat by agriculture and the introduction of herds of domestic cattle. In the bird world rigorous efforts have been made to save the whooping crane, bald-headed vulture, ivory-billed woodpecker and many others to prevent them from following the path to extinction like the passenger-pigeon, great auk and dodo.

Numerous game reserves have been set up all over the world, but these present problems in themselves. In certain areas political pressures are manifest to destroy such important reserves. Even our own government was willing to sacrifice the island of Aldabra, a coral atoll in the Indian Ocean, for an airbase, despite the fact that many important and dwindling species reside there and that some birds, e.g. the frigate birds, would provide a real danger to aircraft through airstrikes. Other reserves are bedevilled by poachers, and species like the rhinoceros have suffered greatly for their aphrodisiac horn and this in spite of the fact that the horn is a thick tuft of hair and has no sexually stimulating properties whatsoever (try munching a mouthful of hair and see!). Finally the problem of over-grazing, starvation and disease have led to increasing awareness of a balanced ecology in the reserves. In Canada, where many wolves were destroyed to allow the Caribou to multiply, these herbivores so overgrazed that many became sickly and diseased and the herds did not flourish until the wolves had been re-introduced to destroy the ailing segment of the stock.

Zoos have a vital part to play and the amorous life of Chi-Chi and Ann-Ann is more than a news-catching gimmick. Giant Pandas are on the verge of extinction. Introduced to the public only at the beginning of this century, they have rapidly become a firm favourite everywhere. So rare are they in their native China bamboo forests that it has been reported that the death penalty exists for the destruction of any member of this species. It is hoped that the successful mating of pandas in zoos will permanently preserve this wonderful animal.

For too long zoos have been regarded simply as places of entertainment. But the modern zoo has important scientific functions to fulfil. There are now about half a million wild vertebrates living in about five hundred zoos and aquaria, and their numbers are increasing. These institutions are continually classifying and storing data on reproduction and gestation, incubation, changes in dentition, physiological and behavioural changes during growth to maturity. Animal diseases and treatments are being studied to provide an immense store of valuable information. Many rare animals have been saved. The classic instance is the Père David's deer, or Mi-Lu, to give it its Chinese name, seen and acquired from the Imperial Hunting Park of Nan-Hai-Tsol (Peking) by Père David, French priest in China, in the year 1865. How it came to be preserved in this park is unknown for it had been extinct for some three thousand years in the wild. In 1905 a flood breached the park wall and all that were not drowned were killed by the starving peasants. Luckily a few survived in Europe, gifts to foreign diplomats. The Eleventh Duke of Bedford, grandfather of the present duke, persuaded the European zoos to let him collect all the available specimens in the park of Woburn Abbey. From eighteen animals they increased to two hundred by 1939 and in 1945, when four hundred deer were thriving, many were distributed to zoos and collections throughout the world. The closest parallel to Père David's deer, of an animal never known to science except in captivity in a park, is provided by the wild white cattle of Chillingham Park in Northumberland. These are thought to be the descendants of the Aurochs or ancient wild ox of Europe. Another mammal that survived in captivity is the Przewalski's horse, discovered in Mongolia in 1879, then the last genuine wild horse in the world. The present world stock is one hundred and ten animals (1967) but some are believed to have been sighted in a remote area in western Mongolia during the summer of 1966. Similarly, the European bison, now extinct in the original wild stock, has continued to multiply; over eight hundred exist today and fifty-seven have been re-introduced to the Bialowieza Forest where they are multiplying successfully. Many animals are now breeding regularly in zoos all over the world and perhaps some, like the tiger (of which there are perhaps only six hundred or so in the wild state today), the gorilla, the European wolf, Grant's zebra and the orang-utan will find a home behind bars in reservations all over the world.

What is the outcome for us all? Perhaps the destruction of species one by one, until it is the turn of man himself to be destroyed in a final, devastating holocaust or is it a reliable population control and survival? What is the fate of the Javan rhino? It may be the ultimate fate of man but that depends on *man*.

THE AGEING PROCESS

WITH THE passage of time all living cells, both plant and animal, undergo structural and functional changes. Some are obvious: the greying of the hair, the lack of co-ordination of the limbs, the tremor on voluntary movement, the failure of sight, etc. Many are so refined and confined to the almost inaccessible interplay of chemical enzymes and sub-microscopic particles in the cells that as yet the mysteries of ageing cannot be unravelled. There is no precise definition of ageing. One concept associates death with a decreased ability of the organism to deal effectively with environmental stresses and strains, due to this cellular alteration. Another hypothesis attributes declining functions of the many organic systems in old age to a loss of cell reproduction, illustrated by the decline in lung, kidney and heart function, etc.

Although there is a great variation in different organs during ageing, a constant decrease of organ function begins about the age of thirty years and gradually continues. Between twenty and eighty the maximum breathing capacity falls by sixty per cent, due to a decreased mobility of the chest wall and related structures. Heart function declines with age and increasing rigidity of the arterial walls and results in an elevation of blood pressure. The speed of nerve conduction falls by fifteen to twenty per cent and muscle strength and co-ordination decrease. (The body musculature diminishes to about one half by eighty years of age, because, unlike most tissues of the body—nervous tissue being another exception

—muscle fibres are unable to reproduce and their numbers remain fixed from birth. As these muscle cells disappear they are replaced by fat and fibrous tissue. Despite exercise there is a loss of strength which is proportional to this decrease in the number of muscle fibres.) The collagen of tendons, ligaments and other tissues, a fibrous protein that constitutes about one third of the body's protein, increases in quantity over the years but becomes more rigid and consequently less elastic, leading to a decrease in pliability of these tissues. Elastic tissue becomes thickened and fragmented and the skin becomes wrinkled and folded, due to this loss of normal elasticity. These changes are due to structural alteration in the proteins themselves, probably by weakening cross linkages or the formation of new linkages among the molecular maze-like configurations.

The bone marrow, the cavity within the bones that produces blood corpuscles of all descriptions, is reduced with ageing, the tissue being replaced by fats. However, the plasma and blood volume (5·5L) show little change with the increase in years and the haemoglobin and total number of blood cells is preserved.

Bones become more brittle and weaker due to alterations in the protein and calcium content. Thus they fracture more easily and heal more slowly. Attempts to stop this osteoporosis by giving calcium, protein diets and vitamin C have not been successful. Collapse of the vertebrae of the cervical and lumbar spine leads to neck ache and arm pains in the former, often called 'fibrositis' of the shoulder, and 'lumbago' (back-ache) and 'sciatica' in the latter.

Of the $12{,}000 \times 10^6$ nerve cells in the adult human brain (a number once again fixed before birth) almost six thousand to seven thousand die each day. Alcohol and other poisons are said to hasten this cell death. However, intellectual performance need not decline with age! The range of information and a detailed working knowledge, often called 'know-how' or 'experience', actually broadens with advancing years. The speed of learning becomes reduced but the correctness and application of the material learned may actually increase. The deliberation of the ageing chess player against his younger, more impulsive opponent is an example that springs readily to mind.

Thus, if the elderly learn less, it is because they often ignore learning, falsely reasoning that new facts and information are beyond their capacity. The mental functions are then no longer exercised and so decline. Many elderly persons continue to exercise the responsibility of important offices with great success but since they are unable to cope with the external mental and physical stresses as well as younger persons there may be a collapse of mental function following illness, change of environment or loss of some close relative.

The older person must cope both physically and psychologically with diminished physical powers outlined above. The body image, imprinted in the parietal lobe of the brain, becomes altered and distorted and a change in environment can precipitate such alterations. For example, old patients, transferred to a hospital, often become very confused, only to return abruptly to normal once they are back at home. There is also the important problem of maintaining self-esteem and position in society; often old people, deficient in physical powers, are classed as spoilt children and lectured to and reprimanded in a fashion that engenders a feeling of inferiority. Slow speech does not necessarily indicate a slow mental outlook, a dribbling mouth senility.

However, when mental deterioration occurs in old age there is usually some gross or microscopic change in the brain structure. The neurones atrophy and the many convolutions of the brain surface flatten out. Insufficient blood flow to the brain leads to a decline in nervous tissue function and mental alterations produce an increased emotional liability (shown by ill temper, pettiness and incongruous remarks and reasoning, depression and lachrymation, i.e. childish behaviour), loss of judgement in social and domestic matters, including

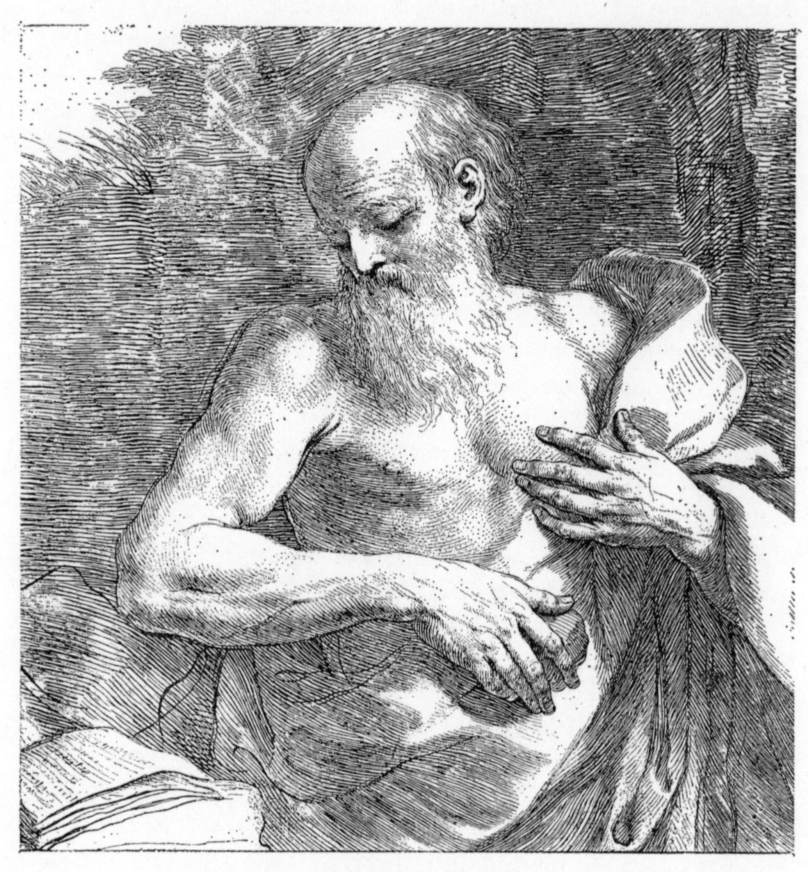

Old Man. *F. Bartolozzi after Guercino*

personal hygiene, varying degrees of loss of recent memory, with only slight loss of remote memory (as shown with persistent recollection of past events) and also occasional confusion, hallucination and fabrications. At their worst these changes are classed as senile dementia (or psychoses) and cerebral arteriosclerosis. The former affects women more than men and in the latter (cerebral arteriosclerosis) the conditions are reversed.

However, an investigation into blood flow and oxygen consumption by cerebral tissue has revealed very little change in the sixty-plus age group, as compared to the twenty-plus age group. Before one can explain the alterations in cerebral function in such a gross manner one must consider the many minor alterations that occur within the cells of the brain, the incorporation of substances like lipofuscin, glycogen, mucoproteins and other 'age pigments' that accumulate in the cells during advancing years, thus altering delicate, interbalanced pathways.

It has been said that in modern society one does not accept or prepare for death during one's lifetime, as was formerly the custom. As age increases there is a greater tendency to avoid confrontation with the idea of death; gradually there may be an increased insecurity and loss of feelings of usefulness and self-confidence. But in many ways nature, by the gradual slowing down of mental and physical processes, prepares us for the inevitable:

Golden lads and girls all must
As chimney-sweepers, come to dust.
Shakespeare.